100 Clinical Cases
and
OSCEs in Medicine

PASTEST
Dedicated to your success

100 Clinical Cases
and
OSCEs in Medicine

David R McCluskey

MD (Hons), FRCP, FRCPI, ILTM

Department of Medicine

Queen's University of Belfast

Belfast

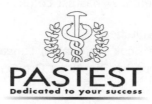

PASTEST
Dedicated to your success

© 2004 PASTEST Ltd
Egerton Court
Parkgate Estate
Knutsford
Cheshire
WA16 8DX

Telephone: 01565 752000

First published 2004

ISBN: 1 904627 12 9

A catalogue record for this book is available from the British Library.

The information contained within this book was obtained by the authors from reliable sources. However, while every effort has been made to ensure its accuracy, no responsibility for loss, damage or injury occasioned to any person acting or refraining from action as a result of information contained herein can be accepted by the publishers or authors.

PasTest Revision Books and Intensive Courses
PasTest has been established in the field of postgraduate medical education since 1972, providing revision books and intensive study courses for doctors preparing for their professional examinations.

Books and courses are available for the following specialties:
MRCGP, MRCP Parts 1 and 2, MRCPCH Parts 1 and 2, MRCPsych, MRCS, MRCOG Parts 1 and 2, DRCOG, FRCA, PLAB Parts 1 and 2.

For further details contact:
PasTest, Freepost, Knutsford, Cheshire WA16 7BR
Tel: 01565 752000   Fax: 01565 650264
www.pastest.co.uk   enquiries@pastest.co.uk

Icons designed by Peter Whitehead
Text prepared by Carnegie Book Production, Lancaster
Printed and bound in Europe by The Alden Group

Contents

Cardiovascular disorders

Respiratory disorders

Gastrointestinal disorders

Haematology

Nervous system

The eye

Endocrinology/metabolic medicine

Musculoskeletal disorders

Dermatology

Renal disorders

Immunology

Acknowledgements

This book is dedicated to my wife Barbara.

I wish to thank Kate Collins, John Collins and Kate Ritchie for helpful advice and suggestions, and David Gill for his expertise in preparing the visual aids. A very special thanks to Eveline Burns for her patience, help, encouragement and expert secretarial skills in the preparation of the text.

About the author

David McCluskey is Head of the Department of Medicine, The Queen's University of Belfast and has over 25 years' experience in undergraduate medical education. He is Consultant Physician to the Royal Victoria Hospital, Belfast, with a special interest in Clinical Immunology. He has written other medical textbooks, including: *Clinical Skills for Medical Students – A Hands-on Guide* (PasTest), *Multiple Choice Questions in Medicine for the MRCP Part 1 Examination*, and *Essential Skills Practice for OSCEs in Medicine*, which can be used in conjunction with this book.

He introduced the OSCE form of assessment into the general medical course for 3rd year students in Belfast in 1996 and has extensive experience in constructing and marking this type of examination, as well as acting as a simulated patient and as an examiner in undergraduate and postgraduate examinations.

Introduction

This book provides all of the essential core information on the most common medical conditions which are used for clinical examination, especially Objective Structured Clinical Examinations (OSCEs) and Practical Assessment of Clinical Examination Skills (PACES).

In these forms of assessment, clinical stations are used. Limited time is available for the candidate to display their knowledge and skills, and it is important that core information is presented to the examiners in a well-structured and efficient manner.

This book describes 100 medical cases which are commonly used in clinical examinations to assess undergraduate medical students and junior doctors training in general medicine. Problem-based cases and specific medical conditions are clearly described, including definitions, classifications and lists of causes, together with all of the essential core knowledge necessary to be successful in clinical examinations.

The cases can be used to revise the main differential diagnoses which must be considered when clinical problems, such as chest pain or shortness of breath, present. They also highlight the key clinical features which occur in specific medical conditions.

This book does not set out to be a comprehensive textbook of medicine but rather should be used along with other medical books. It is designed to be read in conjunction with *Essential Skills Practice for OSCEs in Medicine* by David McCluskey, where candidates can put their clinical skills to the test. Written in a question and answer format, it can be read with a colleague to practice communicating knowledge and skills.

Cardiovascular disorders

CASE 1

The patient with chest pain

Chest pain is one of the most common presenting problems in hospital medical practice. Many of the causes are potentially life-threatening, and therefore chest pain is commonly used in the history-taking part of the examination to assess the ability of the student to take a history which will help to differentiate between the major causes. These can be classified as follows:

1 cardiovascular causes – angina pectoris, myocardial infarction, pericarditis, aortic aneurysm, pulmonary embolism

2 respiratory causes – associated with chest infection, pleurisy, tumours (mesothelioma, bronchogenic carcinoma)

3 musculoskeletal causes – bone, muscle

4 neurological causes – herpes zoster (shingles).

The majority of these topics are covered in the individual case histories. However, it is important to remember a few general points when trying to differentiate between them.

Ask all of the discriminating questions about pain. No matter what part of the body is affected, if a patient complains of pain there are eight features of the pain that must be ascertained. To illustrate this, chest pain is used as an example. By using these discriminating features it is possible to reach a diagnosis relatively easily.

1 **Site.** The patient should be asked about the exact position of the pain – for example whether it is central or peripheral.

2 **Character.** There are many types of pain (sharp, crushing, burning, pressure, crampy, etc). The exact character of the pain often gives an important clue about its cause. Non-verbal cues are also helpful when the patient is asked to describe the type of pain they have been experiencing. Patients use a pointing finger when they mean a sharp pain, a closed fist resting on the sternum when their pain was felt as a pressure or heaviness, or they grip the sides of their chest with their hands and squeeze when the pain is of a tight or crushing nature.

CASE 1

3 **Severity.** It is useful to ask about and document the severity of the pain. This can be done by asking the patient to state on a scale of 0 to 10 how severe the pain felt – where 0 is no pain and 10 is the worst pain the patient has ever experienced.

4 **Radiation.** Pain from internal organs is represented and experienced on the body surface. It often radiates or moves in a characteristic way. For example, renal colic due to a stone in the ureter causes pain in the loin, which radiates around the flank and down into the groin (inguinal region). Pain from the heart is usually felt over the sternum and radiates to the lower jaw and/or down the arms, or it may radiate down only one arm (more commonly the left), while aortic pain may be felt in the back.

5 **Duration.** The patient should be asked to state how long the pain lasted, in minutes or hours. When asked this question patients commonly reply with a vague answer such as 'a long time' or 'quite a while'. This is unhelpful as it is fairly meaningless, so the patient should be politely asked to state in seconds, minutes or hours for how long the longest episode of pain was present. This question is particularly helpful when trying to differentiate between chest pain due to angina pectoris and that due to myocardial infarction. Angina pain seldom persists for more than 20 minutes, whereas the pain of a heart attack usually lasts for more than 30 minutes.

6 **Onset.** Patients should be asked to describe what they were doing or had recently been doing at the time of onset of the pain. Angina pain classically comes on during exercise, but it may occur after a meal, during an argument or awaken the patient from sleep (see angina decubitus). The pain of myocardial infarction more often occurs after exercise or when the patient is at rest.

7 **Exacerbating and relieving factors.** These differ from onset but give similar insight into the cause of pain. The patient should be asked, 'When the pain was present, did you notice anything which you did which made the pain worse or helped to ease the pain?' Angina is made worse by further exercise and is relieved by rest or taking sublingual nitrates. The pain of myocardial infarction does not abate with rest or nitrates and is usually only relieved by opiate analgesics such as morphine or heroin given by injection.

8 **Associated symptoms.** Severe pain by itself can cause the patient to feel nauseated and vomit. Therefore if the patient has these symptoms this gives an indication of pain severity. Chest pain due to angina pectoris is usually less severe and less likely to cause associated symptoms. On the other hand, the severe pain of myocardial infarction is often associated with vomiting. Patients may develop shortness of breath due to the development of venous congestion in the lungs, or they may experience symptoms of sympathetic nervous system over-activity, such as sweating, palpitations and

CASE 1

Cardiovascular disorders

a feeling of panic or impending doom (which is due to the hypotension and shock associated with myocardial muscle necrosis).

With a knowledge of these eight features of chest pain it is possible to differentiate between the major causes and arrive at an accurate diagnosis in most cases. While the classic features of these conditions are described in the case studies, Table 1, on page 7 shows how the discriminating features of chest pain can be used to determine the most likely cause.

Respiratory causes of chest pain

The lung parenchyma has no pain sensory fibres, and therefore pain is only associated with respiratory disease if other tissue is involved.

1 **Tracheitis.** If there is infection or inflammation of the trachea, the patient experiences a sharp retrosternal pain that is associated with and exacerbated by coughing. There may also be other signs of infection, such as fever and purulent sputum.

2 **Pleurisy.** Infection or inflammation of the pleura, which can either occur in isolation or spread from underlying lung disease, causes sharp chest pains that are usually felt in a localised area overlying the area of inflammation. They can vary in severity, are made worse by deep inspiration or coughing, and are eased by splinting the ribs. On auscultation a friction rub is heard over the site of the pain. The rub has a squeaking character, sometimes likened to the noise of chamois leather being rubbed. It is heard during the same phase of inspiration and expiration, is not altered after the patient coughs, and will disappear if an effusion develops as the fluid separates the parietal and visceral layers of the pleura and this prevents them from rubbing together. Pleurisy can be caused by viral or bacterial infection, infiltration with tumours, or granulomatous disease such as sarcoidosis. It can also occur in association with autoimmune disease (eg rheumatoid arthritis).

3 **Tumours.** As mentioned above, tumours can metastasise to the pleura and cause pleuritic pain. Mesothelioma is a primary malignancy that arises in the pleura, is usually slow-growing and is only associated with pain when the tumour begins to erode into the ribs or involve intercostal nerves. The pain is described as a constant 'boring' type of discomfort and is not controlled by simple painkillers. Bronchogenic cancers in the early stages are completely painless and, like mesothelioma, will only cause pain if they spread to involve surrounding tissues such as pleura, ribs, vertebrae, pericardium or intercostal nerves.

CASE
1

Cardiovascular disorders

Musculoskeletal causes of chest pain

Chest pain of musculoskeletal origin is felt as a pleuritic-type pain – that is, it is localised to one area of the chest, it does not radiate, and it is usually made worse by deep inspiration and coughing. The main features that help to differentiate it from pleurisy are as follows:

1   usually there is a history of trauma or exercise which caused the bone damage or caused muscle fibres to tear
2   pain is elicited when the patient uses the muscle groups around the site of pain
3   there is acute local tenderness – a feature that is not usually present in pleurisy.

Neurological causes of chest pain

The commonest neurological cause of chest pain is herpes zoster (shingles). It is felt as a peripheral pain, usually starting in the back and radiating around the side of the chest in the classic unilateral distribution of a dermatome. After four days a vesicular skin eruption appears in the same area and eventually resolves. However, pain and discomfort can persist in this area for up to 2 years (post-herpetic neuralgia) and may be very severe. On examination, areas of depigmentation can often be seen which indicate the site of the previous vesicular eruption.

CASE
1

Table 1 Cardiovascular causes of chest pain

Feature of pain	Angina pectoris	Myocardial infarction	Pericarditis	Aortic aneurysm	Pulmonary embolism
Site	Central chest	Central chest	Central chest	Central chest and back	Peripheral chest
Character	Tightness, crushing weight	Tightness, crushing weight	Sharp, stabbing	Tearing	Sharp
Severity (on a scale of 0–10)	1–5	8–10	1–7	10	2–8
Radiation	Jaw and arms	Jaw and arms	None	Between scapulae at back and down back	None
Duration	< 20 min	> 30 min	Days	Until relieved with strong analgesics	Until relieved
Onset	During exercise, after food, in cold or during stress	After exercise or at rest	No particular time	On or after exercise (increased blood pressure)	No particular time
Relieving factors	Rest, glyceryl trinitrate	Opiates	Simple analgesics	Opiates	Simple analgesics
Associated symptoms	None	Sweating, dyspnoea, nausea and vomiting	Fever	Vomiting, shock, sweating, loss of consciousness	Shortness of breath, haemoptysis

Cardiovascular disorders

CASE 1

Cardiovascular disorders

CASE 2

Angina pectoris

This is a common OSCE history-taking station with a real or simulated patient.

Definition

Angina pectoris is a transient chest pain that is due to myocardial ischaemia brought on by exercise and relieved by rest or sublingual glyceryl trinitrate (GTN).

? Causes

Angina is most commonly caused by arteriosclerosis of one or more of the coronary arteries. It can occur in association with aortic valve disease (see Cases 8 and 9).

Risk factors

These include the following:

- positive family history
- cigarette smoking
- hypertension
- diabetes mellitus
- obesity
- hypercholesterolaemia.

Clinical features

There is episodic central chest pain that is characteristically felt as a tightness or crushing sensation, or as a weight or heaviness. The pain is of variable severity and normally lasts for less than 20 minutes. Acute attacks are relieved by rest or sublingual nitrates. There are five main precipitating causes:

CASE 2

1 **Physical exercise.** The amount of exercise that causes the pain varies from one patient to another and is determined by the severity of the coronary artery narrowing. The distance the patient can walk on the flat or the number of stairs they can climb before the onset of pain is known as their **exercise tolerance**.

2 **Food.** After a meal the metabolic rate increases and there is increased demand for blood flow in the splanchnic circulation. Beware of the overweight businessman who starts to complain of 'indigestion' after meals – it may be postprandial angina.

3 **Stress or emotion.** If individuals with myocardial ischaemia become excited, emotional or stressed, the increased heart rate and peripheral resistance result in increased oxygen demand in the left ventricular muscle.

4 **Cold temperature.** Patients who have angina are more likely to experience episodes of chest pain in cold weather, due to increased peripheral resistance.

5 **Angina decubitus.** Occasionally patients are awakened from sleep by chest pain. This is probably due to an attack of angina being precipitated during rapid eye movement (REM) sleep.

There are no signs specific to angina, but there may be clinical signs present associated with risk factors, such as obesity, hypertension, xanthelasma or clinical features of diabetes.

Investigations

During episodes of pain the ECG will show alterations in the ST segments in the standard and chest leads corresponding to the area of ischaemia. Classically, ST depression of more than 1 mm occurs:

- in leads I and AVL and the V leads if the ischaemia is affecting the anterior wall of the left ventricle
- in leads II, III and AVF if the inferior wall of the ventricle is ischaemic.

Extension of ischaemia into the interventricular septum is indicated by ST-segment depression in V1 to V3, and extension into the lateral wall is indicated by changes in V4 to V6.

Occasionally myocardial ischaemia results in ST-segment elevation in the corresponding leads (Prinzmetal's variant angina) or by T-wave flattening only.

CASE
2

💊 Treatment

1 The patient should be given general advice about reducing risk, such as weight reduction, stopping cigarette smoking and reducing cholesterol levels by switching to a low-fat diet together with lipid-lowering drugs if indicated.

2 Acute attacks can be treated by sublingual nitrates such as GTN tablets or nitrolingual spray.

3 Prophylactic treatment involves the use of three main classes of drugs:

- oral nitrates, such as isosorbide mononitrate. These drugs reduce the peripheral resistance and thus reduce oxygen demand in the cardiac muscle.

- beta-adrenergic blocking drugs (β-blockers). This group of drugs slows the heart rate and reduces the force of contraction of the myocardial muscle fibres (negative inotropic effect). This causes a reduction in the rate and force of contraction of the ventricles and therefore a decrease in oxygen demand.

- calcium-channel blocking drugs. These drugs have a dual action. They mainly reduce peripheral resistance, and some also have a negative inotropic effect on the heart.

Sometimes a single agent is sufficient to control the pain, but often a combination of drugs is required.

At the history-taking station

1 Ask all of the discriminating questions for chest pain (see Case 1).

2 Ask about all of the main risk factors, especially family history.

3 Ask the patient what they are doing to modify their lifestyle and reduce risk factors, such as weight reduction and stopping smoking.

4 Enquire about current drug therapy.

5 Determine whether or not the patient's drug therapy is keeping them pain-free.

CASE
2

CASE 3

Myocardial infarction

This is a common history-taking station with a simulated patient.

📖 Definition

Myocardial infarction occurs when there is an area of myocardial necrosis resulting from an interruption to the blood supply of one or more coronary arteries or their branches.

❓ Causes

It is usually due to thrombosis or embolism from a clot forming on an atheromatous plaque.

📝 Clinical features

There is a sudden onset of severe, crushing, central chest pain that usually lasts for more than 30 minutes (in contrast to angina) and is not relieved by rest or anti-anginal medications. Often there is a past medical history of angina pectoris, as thrombosis is more likely to occur in narrowed coronary arteries and the two conditions share the same risk factors.

The pain may radiate to the arms or lower jaw. It is often associated with sweating, nausea and vomiting, and may cause shortness of breath.

On examination the patient looks shocked and unwell, with an ashen complexion, sweating, and a cold, clammy skin. They usually have a fast, weak pulse and may have a reduced blood pressure and signs of left ventricular failure.

🔍 Investigations

ECG

Classic ECG changes occur in a sequential fashion in the standard and chest leads that correspond to the area of myocardial necrosis (see page 9).

Cardiac enzyme changes

Five enzymes are used as markers of myocardial cell necrosis. The blood level of these enzymes rises in a characteristic pattern following an episode of damage:

- Creatine kinase (muscle/blood isoenzyme) (CKMB). This enzyme is fairly specific to heart muscle cells. The level of CKMB rises rapidly in the blood (within 1–2 hours) but the enzyme quickly disappears from the circulation (levels can normalise within 4–6 hours after the onset of pain). Therefore, although elevation of CKMB activity is a very sensitive and specific test, blood samples need to be obtained within the first few hours after the onset of pain.

- Total creatine kinase (CK). The total level of creatine kinase in the blood is an excellent indicator of myocardial damage. The level of this enzyme reaches a peak within the first 24 hours after an infarction, and returns to normal within 48 hours.

- Aspartate transaminase (AST). This enzyme, which is also released from damaged cardiac cells, reaches a peak level in the serum at 48 hours after an infarction, and returns to normal within 72 hours.

- Lactate dehydrogenase (LDH). This enzyme reaches a peak level in the serum at 72 hours after an infarction, and takes several days to return to normal..

- Troponins. Recently, a number of more specific tests have become available. These involve the measurement of various **troponins**, which are part of the myocardial muscle contractile mechanism. A single blood sample taken 12 hours after the onset of pain is used. If the troponin level is elevated, this indicates that there has been critical ischaemia or necrosis of the cardiac muscle wall. The degree of serum troponin elevation corresponds to the amount of damage.

Classically, the pattern of rise and fall of these enzymes was used to confirm the occurrence of infarction.

CASE
3

Treatment

Adequate pain relief

Patients with myocardial infarction usually require opiate analgesics such as morphine (10–20 mg) or diamorphine (5–10 mg) intravenously, given together with an anti-emetic such as cyclizine (50 mg) to counteract the nausea and vomiting that opiates can induce. The patient should be given oxygen to breathe, and any complications that arise should be quickly identified and treated. Intramuscular injections should be avoided as they would interfere with the CK enzyme results. If you are asked how to treat a myocardial infarction, an excellent answer is, 'Give adequate pain relief, oxygen by inhalation, and treat any complications that may arise.'

Thrombolytic therapy

In the absence of any contraindication (see Table 2), all patients with acute myocardial infarction should be given thrombolytic therapy. The drugs used are either steptokinase or tissue plasminogen activator. Both have been shown to significantly reduce the mortality following myocardial infarction, but are associated with a risk of haemorrhage, especially cerebrovascular bleeding

---

Table 2 Contraindications to thrombolysis

Recent surgery

Active gastrointestinal bleeding or past history of peptic ulceration

Recent head injury

Recent cerebrovascular accident

Streptokinase treatment – should not be used if it has been given within the past 12 months (risk of allergic reaction)

Uncontrolled hypertension

Abdominal aortic aneurysm

Complications

The complications of an infarct can be classified as immediate, early or late, and all of them constitute medical emergencies. Therefore you should have a knowledge of what they are and how they are managed (see Table 3 and the relevant sections in the text).

CASE
3

Table 3 Complications of acute myocardial infarction

Immediate

Asystolic arrest

Ventricular tachycardia

Ventricular fibrillation

Left ventricular failure

Septal rupture

Left ventricular rupture

Acute mitral regurgitation

Haemopericardum

Cardiogenic shock

Early

Left ventricular failure

Arrhythmias – tachycardia, bradycardia, ventricular tachycardia with or without ventricular fibrillation

Left ventricular aneurysm

Late

Left ventricular failure

Aneurysm formation of the ventricle

Ectopic beats

Dressler's syndrome

CASE
3

CASE 4

Ventricular failure

Left ventricular failure

This condition is commonly used in OSCEs for history-taking on shortness of breath and also in X-ray and therapeutics and pharmacology stations.

Definition

It is a condition in which there is impaired function of the left ventricle, resulting in congestion of blood in the pulmonary veins and the development of pulmonary oedema.

Causes

The main causes are:

- ischaemic heart disease
- post-myocardial infarction
- cardiac rhythm disorder
- cardiac valvular disease
- myocarditis
- fluid overload.

Clinical features

The most prominent symptom is dyspnoea due to a combination of pulmonary venous congestion and fluid in the alveoli. The degree and rate of progression of shortness of breath depend on the underlying cause. For example, if there is a sudden onset of ventricular tachycardia or mitral valve rupture, the onset is rapid and the patient becomes very short of breath. If the cause is ischaemic heart disease, the shortness of breath is only noticed on strenuous exertion and it only progresses slowly. Because of compensatory fluid retention and the redistribution of fluid in the pulmonary circulation on lying down, orthopnoea and paroxysmal nocturnal dyspnoea (PND) are usually present.

CASE 4

Although orthopnoea can also occur in respiratory disorders, PND is pathognomonic of left ventricular failure. On clinical examination, the presence of fine crepitations heard at the lung bases and extending up to the mid-zones is characteristic of pulmonary oedema. The higher the level at which crepitations are heard, the greater the severity of pulmonary oedema. In severe cases, pleural effusions may be detected.

Investigations

The most helpful investigation is the chest X-ray, which shows the following four distinct abnormalities and may reveal unilateral (more commonly right-sided) or bilateral pleural effusion:

1 upper lobe venous congestion

2 cardiomegaly

3 interstitial oedema

4 Kerley B lines.

Treatment

Acute attack

Treatment in an acute attack consists of:

1 oxygen by inhalation

2 intravenous diuretics, eg Furosemide (Frusemide) 40–60 mg

3 with or without aminophylline 250 mg by **slow** intravenous injection – provided that the patient is not already on theophylline treatment.

Note: In severe cases which fail to respond to this therapy, removal of 500 ml of blood by venesection can be performed, provided that the patient has a normal haemoglobin level.

CASE
4

Subacute left ventricular failure

1 Diuretic therapy – reduce the fluid load and thereby reduce the amount of work required of the left ventricle. A thiazide or loop diuretic is used, depending on the severity of the condition.

2 Correct any underlying cause, such as a rhythm disturbance.

3 Ensure that there is normal electrolyte balance. When using diuretic drugs it is especially important that the patient does not develop hypokalaemia as a result of potassium loss. Potassium supplements may be necessary.

4 Angiotension-converting enzyme (ACE) inhibitors or ACE-receptor blockers have a central role in the management of heart failure. Their effect is primarily to reduce the pre- and post-load on the heart and thereby reduce the work required of the left ventricle to maintain an adequate cardiac output.

Cardiac asthma

Occasionally patients with left ventricular failure can be mistakenly diagnosed as having acute obstructive airways disease or asthma. This is most likely to occur in patients who develop episodes of paroxysmal nocturnal dyspnoea as the initial or presenting symptom of heart failure. Also, some patients with left-sided failure develop not only pulmonary oedema but also oedema and swelling of the bronchial and bronchiolar mucosa, which results in narrowing of the airways and causes expiratory wheeze. It is therefore understandable that a patient who has acute episodes of dyspnoea in the night and who on auscultation has expiratory wheeze should be considered to be asthmatic. However, these patients fail to respond to bronchodilation therapy, and the use of oral steroids can make the condition worse rather than better, due to the resulting fluid retention. The clinical features that would indicate heart failure would be the presence of fine basal crepitations, a displaced apex beat, a third heart sound (if present), and any signs of right-sided failure. A chest X-ray would show the classic signs of left ventricular failure.

One should always suspect LVF in any middle-aged or elderly patient who develops asthmatic-type symptoms, especially if they fail to show a good response to bronchodilation therapy.

CASE
4

Right ventricular failure

This usually occurs as a consequence of left ventricular failure, and when the two occur together it is termed *congestive cardiac failure*. Sometimes the right ventricle fails as a result of lung disease causing increased resistance to the outflow of blood from that side of the heart. When pulmonary disease is responsible for the right ventricular failure, the condition is termed *cor pulmonale*. In both cases the cause is usually a relatively long-standing condition and there is considerable time for compensatory mechanisms to cause fluid retention. The most prominent symptoms and signs result from fluid overload in the circulation (a raised jugulo-venous pressure). As a result of increased blood volume, raised hydrostatic pressure in vessels and the effect of gravity in the tissues of the lower limbs, patients develop ankle oedema that is worse in the evenings and resolves during each night when they are recumbent (this allows the fluid to be reabsorbed and redistributed in the circulation).

The mainstay of treatment is diuretic therapy to reduce the total blood volume and decrease the volume load, thereby reducing the amount of work required of the right ventricle.

CASE
4

CASE 5

Palpitations and syncopal attacks

This is a relatively common OSCE station used mainly for history taking, although ECGs with common or life-threatening forms of arrhythmias are also used for data interpretation stations.

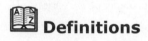 **Definitions**

Palpitations

Palpitations can be defined as the subjective awareness of one's own heart beating. The symptom usually involves a rapid or irregular heartbeat, but there can be a normal or slow heart rate and/or rhythm that is felt to be beating more strongly.

Syncope

Syncope is a sudden loss of consciousness that results from a drop in systolic blood pressure (compare with a fit, drop attack or faint).

? Causes

Syncopal attacks are precipitated by anything that reduces the systolic blood pressure, thereby causing impaired blood flow to the brain. They may be due to a rapid, slow or irregular pulse which can be experienced as palpitations before the patient loses consciousness.

At some time in their life everyone experiences the subjective feeling of their heart beating, eg after strenuous exercise. These are physiological palpitations, and they can also occur in people who are anxious or nervous. It is important to be able to differentiate between physiological (harmless) and pathological palpitations. Pathological palpitations may lead to more serious or life-threatening arrhythmias and require medical treatment.

Cardiovascular disorders

✍ Features of physiological palpitations

These palpitations are usually fast and regular in rhythm. They gradually increase in rate until they reach a maximum, and when they abate they do so gradually. Although they may be associated with feelings of anxiety, such as tremor and sweating, the blood pressure is maintained and they do not usually cause loss of consciousness, chest pain or shortness of breath. During an episode the ECG rhythm is invariably sinus tachycardia.

✍ Features of pathological palpitations

These palpitations may be associated with a slow, fast or irregular rate and rhythm. They often commence and terminate abruptly. They are more likely to be associated with symptoms of dizziness, chest pain, shortness of breath or syncope. A variety of cardiac rhythm disorders can cause palpitations.

Atrial fibrillation

When the rate is rapid, atrial fibrillation is experienced as an irregular beating in the chest, and is often described by the patient as feeling like a frightened bird fluttering in a cage. The condition usually responds to digoxin or amiodarone therapy, but sometimes requires DC cardioversion to restore sinus rhythm.

Many other arrhythmias cause palpitations. These include atrial flutter, supraventricular tachycardias of various types, eg Wolff-Parkinson-White syndrome, ventricular ectopics and self-terminating ventricular tachycardias.

CASE
5

CASE 6

Mitral stenosis

This type of case is used in the clinical examination station, as some older patients with stenosis are readily available to be used as patients in examinations.

Definition

Mitral stenosis is a narrowing of the mitral valve and is usually a sequel to rheumatic fever. It is more common in women than in men, with a female:male ratio of 2:1.

Clinical features

The clinical features usually appear in early adult life, approximately 10–12 years after an attack of rheumatic fever. The onset is characterised by shortness of breath on exertion, which gradually becomes more severe. Patients often develop atrial fibrillation in association with the stenotic valve. This may be paroxysmal at first, but eventually it becomes persistent.

Occasionally patients describe haemoptysis, which is due to rupture of small distended endobronchial blood vessels. There is also an increased risk of recurrent respiratory infection, as the congested oedematous lungs are more prone to bacterial infection.

On clinical examination, inspection of the patient may reveal a classic malar flush that is characterised by small distended capillaries (which are often slightly cyanosed) over the cheeks and the chin. The pulse is small-volume, and on auscultation of the heart there is a loud first heart sound and a normal second heart sound, followed quickly by the opening snap. There is a mid- to late diastolic murmur, and if the patient is in sinus rhythm the murmur becomes louder just before the first heart sound. This accentuation of the murmur is due to left atrial contraction, and is absent in patients who have associated atrial fibrillation.

Cardiovascular disorders

The severity of the murmur is inversely proportional to the interval between the second heart sound and the opening snap. In other words, the shorter the interval between the second heart sound and the opening snap, the greater the pressure in the left atrium must be, and therefore the more severe the stenosis. The loudness of the murmur has little to do with the severity of the stenosis, although the length of the murmur does correlate with severity to some degree.

Treatment

Treatment includes prophylactic antibiotic therapy prior to any procedure, to prevent bacterial endocarditis. Atrial fibrillation, if present, should be treated with digoxin, and any cardiac failure that is present should be treated. Patients should undergo echocardiography to assess the severity of the stenosis, and should be considered for valvotomy or mitral valve replacement surgery if necessary.

CASE
6

CASE 7

Mitral incompetence

This common cardiac valvular defect is frequently used in clinical examinations.

Definition

Mitral incompetence is a cardiac valvular defect in which the mitral valve allows blood to regurgitate into the left atrium during systole.

Clinical features

This defect is more common in men than in women, and it may be secondary to left ventricular failure with dilatation of the mitral valve ring, or a consequence of rheumatic heart disease, a complication of myocardial infarction or due to ischaemic heart disease causing papillary muscle dysfunction.

The clinical features are increasing shortness of breath on exertion, usually occurring gradually over a long period of time unless the cause of the incompetence is an acute event, such as acute papillary muscle dysfunction or myocardial infarction. On examination the patient will have a large pulse pressure, atrial fibrillation is common, and the apex beat will be displaced towards the axilla due to dilatation of the left ventricle. A palpable systolic thrill may be felt over the apex, and there will be a pansystolic murmur, best heard at the apex and radiating to the left axilla, increasing in loudness on expiration. The first heart sound will be soft due to failure of closure of the mitral valve, and a third heart sound may be present.

The diagnosis can be confirmed by echocardiography, and a chest X-ray will show the characteristic features of left ventricular failure (see page 16).

Treatment

Medical therapy involves treating any left ventricular failure or rhythm disturbance that is present, and the use of prophylactic antibiotics to prevent bacterial endocarditis. For severe cases, valve replacement is required.

CASE 8

Aortic stenosis

📖 Definition

This is defined as a narrowing of the aortic valve. Around 50% of cases occur in bicuspid aortic valves that become calcified, and 50% as a sequel to rheumatic fever where the disease process involves the normal tricuspid valve. This condition is more common in men than in women, with a male:female ratio of 3:1. It usually presents in people over the age of 50 years.

📝 Clinical features

The symptoms that occur in this condition are due to decreased cardiac output causing weakness of the skeletal muscles, as well as tiredness. Angina pectoris, syncopal attacks on exertion and symptoms of left ventricular failure may also occur.

The first symptom that patients often describe is general tiredness and reduced exercise capacity, due to the obstruction of outflow from the left ventricle causing a reduced cardiac output to muscles. The continued obstruction to outflow of the left ventricle causes left ventricular hypertrophy. This increase in muscle mass in the left ventricle, together with the reduced coronary artery filling time in diastole, results in the development of symptoms of coronary artery insufficiency or angina pectoris.

Patients can sometimes have syncopal attacks, which are due to transient episodes of hypotension. Although the exact cause of these is unknown, it may be related to outflow obstruction in the stenosed valve, possibly due to transient arrhythmias causing a drop in blood pressure, or due to abnormal control of blood pressure by the baroreceptors in patients with reduced systolic outflow pressure.

The development of left ventricular failure is a sinister sign in aortic stenosis. Once patients develop symptoms of pulmonary oedema with shortness of breath, orthopnoea and paroxysmal nocturnal dyspnoea, the stenosis is so severe that the left ventricle is incapable of maintaining the cardiac output. Occasionally, sudden death can occur due to arrhythmia.

CASE
8

Cardiovascular disorders

On clinical examination, the characteristic signs are as follows:

- there is a low-volume pulse with a small pulse pressure
- the pulse is plateau in character
- a systolic thrill may be palpable at the apex or over the aortic area
- the apex beat is thrusting in character due to the left ventricular hypertrophy, but if failure has developed the left ventricle dilates and the apex beat is displaced towards the axilla
- the second heart sound is diminished in character
- the most prominent sign is an ejection systolic murmur, which may be heard loudest at the apex but is always heard in the aortic area, and which radiates up the neck on the right side. The murmur is increased on expiration
- a fourth heart sound may be present
- the characteristic murmur is a harsh crescendo–decrescendo murmur.

Investigations

On ECG there will be marked left ventricular hypertrophy, and left bundle branch block may be present. Chest X-ray may show evidence of calcification of the aortic valve cusps or valve ring, with some post-stenotic dilatation of the aorta. If left ventricular failure has developed, the classic signs will be present on the X-ray.

Echocardiography will confirm the diagnosis and may also give some indication as to the severity of the stenosis. Cardiac catheterisation may be necessary to confirm severe aortic stenosis and identify the pressure gradient across the valve.

Treatment

If left untreated, severe aortic stenosis has a poor prognosis, with an average life expectancy of less than two years. It is therefore important to treat any cardiac failure that is present, to treat symptoms of angina and to refer the patient for surgical assessment with a view to aortic valve replacement.

CASE
8

CASE 9

Aortic incompetence

This condition is frequently used in clinical examination stations, when the student is asked to feel the pulse and auscultate the heart.

Definition

Aortic incompetence is a condition in which the aortic valve fails to close completely during diastole, and blood regurgitates from the aorta back into the left ventricle.

? Causes

There are four main underlying causes of this condition:

1 severe or prolonged hypertension
2 damage to the aortic valve in rheumatic fever
3 infection of the rheumatic valve (most notably bacterial endocarditis or syphilis)
4 in association with connective tissue disease, particularly rheumatoid arthritis or Marfan's syndrome.

Clinical features

The clinical features result from the combined increase in pressure and volume load on the left ventricle with increased oxygen requirement of the left side of the heart.

Shortness of breath is the most prominent symptom, and this is due to left ventricular failure. Angina pectoris usually develops approximately two years after the onset of exertional dyspnoea. Patients may have symptoms or signs of the underlying cause.

On clinical examination there are several signs which may classically be present in association with this condition:

1 the pulse is of a collapsing (water-hammer) nature
2 there are prominent carotid pulsations (Corrigan's sign)

CASE
9

Cardiovascular disorders

3 there is a wide pulse pressure

4 digital pulsation can be detected, as can capillary pulsation as visualised by applying partial pressure to the nail and observing the capillaries in the nail bed (Quincke's sign)

5 on auscultation of the heart the first sound is normal in character, but the second heart sound is soft due to the absence of the aortic component

6 there is an early diastolic murmur, which is best heard at the left sternal edge and is loudest when the patient holds their breath in expiration

7 a third heart sound may be present if left ventricular failure is present, and a fourth heart sound may also be present

8 an Austin Flint murmur may be present (this is a diastolic rumbling murmur which is heard at the apex and is due to turbulence of blood flow at the mitral valve).

Auscultating over the femoral arteries may elicit two clinical signs:

1 Duroziez' sign. If pressure is applied distally with the bell of the stethoscope over the femoral artery, a soft diastolic murmur may be heard. This is due to regurgitation of blood in the femoral artery during diastole.

2 Pistol-shot femorals. On auscultation over the femoral artery with the diaphragm of the stethoscope, 'pistol-shot' sounds may be heard with each systole.

Investigations

The ECG may show evidence of left ventricular hypertrophy, there may be left axis deviation, and a left bundle branch block pattern may be present. Chest X-ray may reveal cardiac enlargement and other signs of left ventricular failure. The diagnosis is confirmed by echocardiography and/or cardiac catheterisation.

Treatment

Medical therapy involves the treatment of any underlying cause, if present. Treat the patient for angina pectoris or cardiac failure if either of these is present, and consider referral for surgical replacement of the diseased valve.

Patients with aortic incompetence also have a reduced life expectancy. If untreated, most patients will succumb to the disease within 10 years.

CASE
9

Cardiovascular disorders

CASE 10

Pulmonary valve disease

✎ Clinical features

Pulmonary valve diseases are rare, although occasionally patients may have increased blood flow through a normal valve that causes a soft systolic murmur. True pulmonary stenosis is most commonly a congenital condition which causes a harsh murmur.

The most prominent symptom of pulmonary stenosis is shortness of breath on exertion. On auscultation there is a harsh ejection systolic murmur heard at the second interspace on the left side of the chest in the mid-clavicular line. The second heart sound is widely split due to delayed closure of the pulmonary valve.

Pulmonary incompetence is extremely rare. It may occur as a consequence of pulmonary valve infection due to bacterial endocarditis, which is more likely to occur in intravenous drug users. The symptoms are shortness of breath on exertion together with symptoms and signs of the underlying cause.

On examination, an early diastolic murmur is heard at the left sternal edge, and the intensity of the murmur is increased during the inspiratory phase of respiration. The pulmonary component of the second heart sound is diminished.

The main diagnostic tests for pulmonary valve disease are echocardiography and cardiac catheterisation of the right side of the heart.

⬤ Treatment

Treatment of these valve conditions necessitates cardiac surgery with replacement or reconstruction of the diseased valve.

CASE 10

CASE 11

Tricuspid valve disease

Clinical features

Primary tricuspid valve disease, like pulmonary valve disease, is extremely uncommon, although it can occur as a consequence of rheumatic heart disease or bacterial endocarditis, or as a congenital condition. Tricuspid incompetence secondary to congestive heart failure is quite common, due to the dilatation of the right ventricle that occurs in this condition.

Tricuspid valve conditions cause shortness of breath on exertion as the most prominent symptom, and may lead to secondary left ventricular failure.

Tricuspid stenosis is very uncommon. It causes a loud first heart sound, and a late diastolic murmur which is heard best over the tricuspid area of the precordium, the murmur being increased on inspiration.

Tricuspid incompetence results in a soft first heart sound, and a pansystolic murmur that is heard best over the tricuspid area of the precordium. Due to the backflow of blood into the right atrium and increasing pressure in the jugular venous system, giant V-waves occur in the jugular venous pulse, and due to the increased pressure during systole, which is transmitted to the inferior vena caval system, a pulsatile liver may be felt. This is best detected by bimanual palpation of the liver. With each heartbeat the liver is felt to expand between the palpating hands.

Tricuspid valve disease is best diagnosed by echocardiography and right-sided cardiac catheterisation.

Treatment

The underlying cause should be treated if possible. If the degree of valve damage is severe, valve replacement may be necessary.

Cardiovascular disorders

CASE 12

Pulmonary embolism and deep venous thrombosis

Pulmonary embolism

This is an acute medical emergency, and all students are expected to know how to diagnose and manage it. It would be unusual to have a real patient with this condition, and it is more likely that a simulated patient with a history suggestive of a small or medium-sized pulmonary embolism would be encountered in the examination.

Definition

Pulmonary embolism is defined as impaction in the pulmonary vascular bed of a portion of a detached thrombus or foreign matter, resulting in infarction of the lung tissue.

Around 90% of cases occur as a complication of deep venous thrombosis, but other tissue or matter (eg amniotic fluid, fat, air, bone marrow, fragments of tumour) can act as emboli, and occasionally emboli may arise in the right side of the heart due to cardiac failure, atrial fibrillation or bacterial endocarditis affecting either the tricuspid valve or the pulmonary valve.

Clinical features

The clinical features are predominantly cardiovascular and depend mainly on the size of the embolus. They can be considered in three main groups, namely massive, moderate and small pulmonary embolism.

Massive pulmonary embolism

This affects more than 50% of the pulmonary arterial circulation, and causes sudden onset of chest pain, shortness of breath and signs of acute right ventricular failure. The patient will have reduced blood pressure, and they may lose consciousness and have tachycardia. If left untreated, death will usually result within two hours.

CASE 12

On clinical examination, the patient will be unconscious and cyanosed, with a tachycardia and low or unrecordable blood pressure. There will be pulsation evident in the second interspace in the mid-clavicular line, a loud pulmonary second heart sound will be heard and the jugular venous pressure will be raised.

Moderate pulmonary embolism

This causes less than 50% occlusion of the pulmonary artery system. Moderately sized embolism usually presents with symptoms of sudden onset of shortness of breath, cough and haemoptysis. Shortly after the onset, pleuritic-type chest pain may develop and on clinical examination there will be tachycardia and raised jugular venous pressure with a positive hepatojugular reflux and a loud pulmonary second heart sound. A pleural rub may be audible (although this can take some time to develop). The blood pressure may be low if the area of infarction is large, and the patient may be cyanosed.

Small pulmonary embolism

Patients may simply describe a transient episode of sharp pleuritic-type chest pain, cough with or without haemoptysis and transient dyspnoea. On clinical examination, little may be found, although during the acute episode the patient might have a slight tachycardia. The majority of patients with pulmonary embolism will show evidence of deep venous thrombosis in the legs, although in some cases the thrombosis may not be obvious, as it may involve the pelvic venous system.

Diagnosis

Chest X-ray is often normal or may show an area of wedge-shaped infarct of the lung tissue distal to the thrombosis. There may be a small pleural effusion on the affected side. In patients who have had multiple small pulmonary emboli, previous areas of plate atelectasis may be apparent or the diaphragm may be elevated on the affected side. The ECG may show changes of a deep S wave in standard lead I, a pathological Q-wave and T wave inversion in standard lead III, and evidence of right bundle branch block. However, these ECG changes are not always present, particularly in patients with a small or moderately sized embolism.

The best diagnostic tests are spiral CT scanning of the lungs or pulmonary angiography. Ventilation-perfusion scans in the acute phase may show an area of lung tissue that is ventilated but not perfused (this is termed a mismatch). However, if the test is delayed for more than 48 hours the resorption of air and collapse in the affected part of the lung will convert to a matched defect, which is indistinguishable from that seen with other forms of lung disease.

Cardiovascular disorders

CASE
12

Treatment

The treatment of this condition depends very much on its severity. For patients who are hypotensive and unconscious, urgent treatment is required to raise the blood pressure and to remove or redissolve the clot. This may require embolectomy or thrombolysis. For patients with less life-threatening embolism, the treatment is anticoagulation with intravenous heparin or subcutaneous low-molecular-weight heparin for seven days followed by oral anticoagulation using warfarin for a period of six months.

Deep venous thrombosis

This is a common condition that can occur in hospitalised patients, and all junior house officers would be expected to be competent in its diagnosis and management. For this reason, it would commonly be encountered at a clinical examination station using either a real patient or photographs of a single swollen leg.

Definition

Deep venous thrombosis is the presence of a blood clot in a deep vein, most commonly one of the deep veins of the lower limbs, although it also occurs in pelvic vessels and may rarely occur in the upper limbs.

Clinical features

A blood clot is prone to develop in a vein if one or more of the following three abnormalities occur:

1 changes in the constituents of the blood, that promote coagulation

2 alteration in the rate of flow of blood, that allows stasis

3 abnormalities in the vessel wall.

The commonest cause of deep venous thrombosis is immobility. It occurs particularly in individuals who sit for prolonged periods in a cramped position, such as when making a prolonged journey by air or car. It also occurs in individuals who are bed-bound, and is particularly common in patients after surgical procedures or myocardial infarction. This is because during these events there is an increase in the levels of the acute-phase reactants of the blood, especially fibrinogen, which further increases the risk of clot formation. Patients with thrombophilia, polycythaemia, myeloma or Waldenström's macroglobulinaemia are all at increased risk of clotting in veins. Any inflammation or tumour infiltration of the veins, or any pressure from outside the venous system, pressing on the vein, may also increase the risk of clot formation.

CASE
12

The symptoms that the patient experiences will be swelling of one leg, and pain (usually in the calf of the leg) which is worse on weight-bearing.

On examination there will be obvious swelling of the limb, which can be recorded as an increase in diameter around the calf muscle or the thigh compared with the other limb. The temperature of the affected limb will be increased, and it will feel warm to the touch. The skin may have a dusky red discoloration, and there will be pitting oedema of the foot and ankle. On palpation of the calf muscle, tenderness may be elicited, and a clot can sometimes be felt in the popliteal vein. Tapping lightly over the tibia will elicit pretibial tenderness. On dorsiflexion of the foot, pain or discomfort will be experienced in the calf region. However, this sign should be elicited with caution, as repeated dorsiflexion will compress the vein and may dislodge a further small portion of clot to become an embolus.

The diagnosis is confirmed by Doppler venography or venogram using contrast which will demonstrate clot in the affected deep veins.

Treatment

Treatment consists of subcutaneous low-molecular-weight heparin for the acute phase (4–5 days) plus pain relief, and the patient should then be commenced on oral anticoagulation with the aim of achieving an international normalised ratio (INR) of 3. Treatment should continue for a period of three months and can then be discontinued. Any underlying cause of the condition should be sought and treated. Recurrent deep vein thromboses should be thoroughly investigated for evidence of a clotting disorder or underlying malignancy.

CASE 13

The abnormal pulse

Because there are many patients in the community with heart disease, it is relatively easy to ask one who has an abnormal pulse to allow a number of students to feel the pulse and discuss its diagnosis and management.

The pulses that are commonly used in the OSCE include the following:

- atrial fibrillation
- plateau pulse
- collapsing pulse
- bradycardia
- ectopic beats.

Before discussing each of these, it is worth recalling the important aspects to note about any pulse. At an OSCE station where you may be asked to feel a pulse, be sure to work through this method of reporting to demonstrate that you have a system for assessing the pulse.

First, feel both radial pulses to ensure that they are synchronous and of equal volume. If they are not, the patient has either coarctation of the aorta or a dissecting aneurysm. If they are, then feel one radial pulse and note the following:

1 **Rate.** Measured in beats per minute.

2 **Rhythm.** Is it regular or irregular? If it is irregular, is the rhythm regularly irregular (ie with a pattern to the irregularity) or irregularly irregular (ie with no discernible pattern)?

3 **Volume.** Is the pulse volume normal, low or high? Is the volume the same for each beat?

4 **Character.** There are only four pulse characters with which you need to be concerned. See page 35.

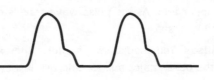

(a) normal

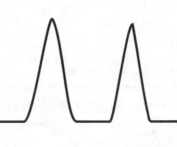

(b) collapsing   Aortic incompetence

(c) plateau   Aortic stenosis

(d) bisferiens   Aortic stenosis and
                                                              incompetence

5 Vessel wall. Is the wall of the artery palpable or not? A normal artery wall
cannot be felt. If the artery feels like a piece of cord, the patient has
arteriosclerosis. If you wish to search for other evidence of this, ask for
permission to look at the medial aspect of the upper arm with the patient
holding their elbow flexed to 90°. If there is significant arteriosclerosis of the
brachial artery, with each heartbeat a snake-like movement will be seen to
travel down towards the antecubital fossa. This physical sign is called
locomotor brachialis, and it occurs because the brachial artery is fixed at a
point in the axilla and in the antecubital fossa. Any thickening and
elongation results in the artery adopting a tortuous course along the medial

CASE
13

aspect of the upper arm. As the pulse wave travels down the artery, the latter wriggles like a snake.

6 **Peripheral pulses.** You should always inform the examiner that you would normally feel the other major pulses, and ask if they wish you to proceed. If they do, feel both carotids, the femorals, popliteals, posterior tibial and dorsalis pedis, and comment on their presence or absence and the symmetry of pulse volume.

Atrial fibrillation

This pulse is irregularly irregular, and the irregularity is in both rhythm and pulse volume. The common causes are ischaemic heart disease, rheumatic heart disease, mitral valve disease and thyrotoxicosis, but atrial fibrillation can also occur in hypertensive heart disease, as a complication of myocardial infarction and as a result of alcohol-induced cardiomyopathy.

The true heart rate can only be determined accurately at the apex, as some of the very weak ventricular contractions do not get transmitted down the radial artery to the wrist. The difference in pulse rate between the apex of the heart and the radial artery is called the **pulse deficit**. The aim of therapy in atrial fibrillation is to restore sinus rhythm. If this is not possible, the objective is to maintain the apical rate at less than 100 beats per minute.

Plateau pulse

This type of pulse is found in patients with aortic stenosis. Once felt it should alert you to remember the features of the heart sounds and murmur found in this disorder (see Case 8), as frequently the examiner's next instruction is, 'Now listen to this patient's heart and tell me what you hear.'

Collapsing (water-hammer) pulse

This is a large-volume pulse that strikes the palpating fingers forcefully. It is best elicited by placing the examining hand across the flexor aspect of the patient's wrist so that the radial artery runs transversely across your palm. Elevate the patient's arm so that their hand is well above the level of their heart.

If a collapsing pulse is present, you will feel a more forceful pulse hitting the palm of your examining hand. The pulse is not sustained, and each pulse wave is shorter than normal.

CASE
13

Cardiovascular disorders

This type of pulse is one of the many classic features of aortic incompetence (see Case 9). After finding such a pulse you will almost certainly be asked to auscultate the heart and report your findings. You may even be asked to name all the other signs of aortic incompetence – so be prepared!

Bradycardia

This is defined as a heart rate of less than 60 beats per minute. It can occur in normal people with no underlying disease, and is especially common in very fit young people. Other causes of bradycardia include the following:

- drugs, especially β-blockers
- hypothyroidism
- hypothermia
- an early complication of a posterior myocardial infarction
- complete heart block – in this case the pulse is 40 beats per minute and fails to increase with exercise.

Ectopic beats

Many people have occasional extrasystoles, but they occur more often in patients with ischaemic heart disease or following a myocardial infarction, when an area of scar tissue can act as an electrical focus for ectopic beats. On feeling the pulse the basic rhythm is regular, but there will be an extra one or more pulse beats every minute, sometimes associated with a compensatory pause. Usually ectopic beats are benign and require no treatment.

Indications for therapy with anti-arrhythmic drugs include the following:

- frequent ectopics
- runs of ectopics (three or more occurring together)
- episodes of ventricular tachycardia or ventricular fibrillation triggered by ectopics.

CASE
13

CASE 14

The patient with raised jugular venous pressure

This is a common clinical examination station. Many patients are available who have mild to moderate right ventricular failure and are willing to be used in clinical examinations. From the examiners' point of view this station is excellent as it can be used to test knowledge of surface anatomy and of the physiology of the cardiac cycle, students' awareness of a number of serious medical conditions associated with a raised jugular venous pressure, and their ability to elicit and interpret a clinical sign.

Definition

This condition is defined as increased pressure in the jugular venous system.

Fig 1 Anatomy of the jugular venous system.

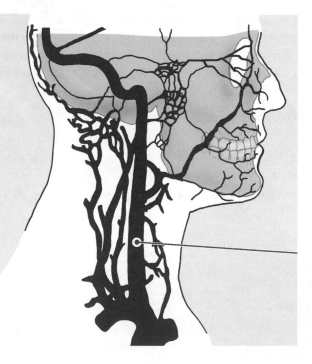

Internal jugular vein (runs behind the sternomastoid muscle)

CASE 14

When judging whether or not these veins are distended with blood, it is necessary to place the patient in a recumbent position with the upper half of their body at 45° to the horizontal (see fig 2). This ensures that in a normal person the right atrium is at the level of the angle of Louis (the sternomanubrial joint), and there should be no column of blood distending the right-sided jugular veins above the level of the clavicle. If blood **is** distending the veins this indicates increased pressure within the right atrium, and the vertical height of the upper level of blood in the jugular vein is directly proportional to the pressure in the atrium.

Since the internal jugular vein is directly in line with the superior vena cava, this is the best vessel to use. However, since this vessel runs posterior and lateral to the sternomastoid muscle it is less easily seen than the external jugular vein.

Fig 2

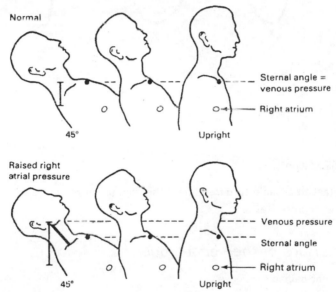

? Causes

Causes of distended jugular veins include the following:

- right ventricular cardiac failure
- tricuspid incompetence
- fluid overload
- superior vena caval obstruction
- raised intrathoracic pressure
- constrictive pericarditis
- pericardial effusion.

CASE 14

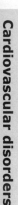

Venous pulsation

If the veins are distended, they display a characteristic double waveform with each cardiac cycle, which is related to the pressure transmitted from the contracting right atrium and right ventricle.

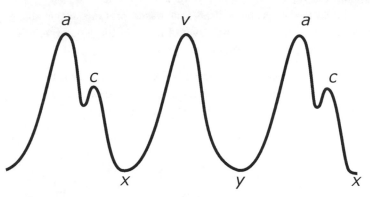

a: atrial contraction

x: atrial relaxation

v: ventricular contraction

c: tricuspid valve closure

y: ventricular filling

It is important to be able to differentiate the various pulse waves from the nearby carotid arterial pulse wave.

Characteristics of the venous pulse:

- is not palpable
- varies with position
- usually has an upper level
- can be obliterated by pressure
- normally has two waveforms
- increases on inspiration.

Characteristics of the arterial pulse:

- is palpable
- does not change with position

CASE 14

Cardiovascular disorders

- has no upper level
- is not easily obliterated
- has a single waveform
- does not change with respiration.

Abnormal waveforms

- No *a*-waves – atrial fibrillation.
- Giant *a*-waves – due to right atrial hypertrophy, and may be seen in patients with tricuspid stenosis, pulmonary stenosis or pulmonary hypertension.
- Cannon waves – the term given to intermittent giant *a*-waves. They occur in complete heart block due to the fact that occasionally the right atrium contracts when the tricuspid valve is closed. All the pressure of the atrial contraction is transmitted to the venous drainage system.
- Giant *v*-waves – these occur in patients with tricuspid incompetence, ie the right ventricular systolic pressure is transmitted back into the right atrium and directly into the jugular venous system.

The hepatojugular reflux

This is an extremely useful adjunctive clinical test that is used in patients with an elevated jugular venous pressure or suspected right ventricular failure.

Method:

1 Ask the patient if they have any abdominal tenderness. If they have, do not proceed. Otherwise, continue with the following steps.

2 Explain that you are going to apply pressure to their abdomen by pressing firmly with your hand.

3 Instruct the patient to continue to breathe normally throughout the procedure.

As a result of increasing the intra-abdominal pressure, blood is forced out of the mesenteric veins via the portal vein into the inferior vena cava and on to the right heart chambers. Normally this increased volume of blood will be pumped out into the pulmonary arterial circulation within five heartbeats. If the right ventricle is incapable of dealing with the increased volume load, blood accumulates in the right atrium and the veins draining into the atrium. By a combination of the jugular venous pressure and the hepatojugular reflux it is possible to assess the function of the right ventricle and differentiate between the causes of an elevated jugular venous pressure.

CASE
14

Assessment of right ventricular function

A patient with a right ventricle on the verge of failure (incipient right ventricular failure) would have a jugular venous pressure of zero but a positive hepatojugular reflux, ie the right ventricle would not be able to cope with an increased fluid load, and when it was given more blood to pump there would be a rise in the jugular venous pressure.

Differentiation between the causes of a raised jugular venous pressure

In a patient with an elevated jugular venous pressure, by observing the venous waves and using the hepatojugular reflux it is possible to differentiate between some of the causes of a raised jugular venous pressure.

To understand this it is important to remember the following:

1 if there is an obstruction to the superior vena cava, the normal waveforms originating in the heart or any increased pressure in the right atrium (such as occurs with a positive hepatojugular reflux) cannot be transmitted to the jugular venous system

2 if there is reduced filling of the cardiac chambers, there will be a resultant reduction in stroke volume and pressure.

Therefore:

- in right ventricular failure the jugular venous pressure is elevated but varies with position; the hepatojugular reflux is positive; and waveforms are normal.

- in superior vena cava obstruction the jugular venous pressure is elevated, the upper level cannot be ascertained and the degree of distension does not vary with position; the hepatojugular reflux does not increase pressure within the veins; and no waveforms are present.

- in constructive pericarditis or pericardial effusion the jugular venous pressure is raised and varies with position; the hepatojugular reflux is positive; and the waveforms show a greatly decreased amplitude.

**CASE
14**

CASE 15

Examination of swollen leg(s)

This is a relatively common clinical examination station or clinical sign (photograph) station.

Unilateral swollen leg

The differential diagnosis is deep venous thrombosis, ruptured Baker's cyst or cellulitis.

Deep venous thrombosis

This is dealt with in detail elsewhere (see Case 12).

Ruptured Baker's cyst

This occurs when a popliteal cyst ruptures and synovial fluid tracks down the leg into the calf muscles. A popliteal cyst is an outpouch of the synovial membrane of the knee joint which protrudes through a posterior rupture of the knee-joint capsule.

Clinical features

This condition may mimic an acute deep venous thrombosis with pain and swelling in the calf that is worse on weight-bearing, and tenderness on palpation. The leg is swollen, but there is no venous congestion and no pretibial tenderness.

Investigations

Rule out deep vein thrombosis by using Doppler venography or venogram. Injection of contrast material into the knee joint and X-ray will reveal contrast escaping out of the joint space into the popliteal fossa.

Treatment

Bed rest and analgesia are usually sufficient, as the rupture often heals spontaneously. Occasionally surgery is required.

CASE 15

Cellulitis (also known as erysipelas)

Although this condition can occur in any part of the body, it commonly affects a lower limb and presents as unilateral swelling of a leg.

Definition

Cellulitis consists of infection spreading in the skin and subcutaneous tissues that can result in swelling due to oedema and lymphoedema.

? Causes

Beta-haemolytic streptococcal organisms are the commonest cause, and an abrasion, cut or local trauma is often found close to the area of infection. Staphylococcal infection can also result in cellulitis, but is less common.

Clinical features

There is an area of inflamed skin that is usually well demarcated, and the area is painful, tender, swollen and feels hot to the touch. There may be evidence of ascending lymphangitis with red lines travelling up towards the groin on the affected side, together with painful tender regional lymph node enlargement. The patient usually feels generally unwell, with malaise and fever.

Investigations

There is pyrexia, and a raised total white cell count due to a neutrophilia. Skin swabs may identify the offending streptococcal organism or, if the patient has a spiking fever, blood cultures may be positive.

Treatment

Treatment consists of benzylpenicillin administered intravenously until the infection is under control, and then penicillin V or flucloxacillin given orally for 7–10 days. Patients who are allergic to penicillin should be treated with a macrolide antibiotic.

Bilateral leg swelling

The commonest cause of bilateral swelling of the lower limbs is oedema due to right ventricular failure. Other causes include myxoedema and lymphoedema.

Oedema

A number of medical conditions can result in the accumulation of oedema fluid in the

CASE
15

Cardiovascular disorders

dependent parts of the body, resulting in swelling of the feet, ankles and lower legs. The swelling gets worse as the day progresses, due to the action of gravity, and resolves during the night.

? Causes

1   Right ventricular failure

2   Any cause of hypoproteinaemia:

- Renal disease

- Malabsorption

- Protein-losing enteropathy

- Liver disease.

3   Fluid overload.

Treatment

Treat the underlying cause and give diuretics with or without salt-free albumin infusion if the cause is a low serum protein level.

Localised myxoedema

This causes bilateral swelling of the legs due to the accumulation of mucopolysaccharides, especially in the pretibial region of the legs, and it can extend into the dorsum of the feet and toes. It is non-pitting and occurs in patients with hypothyroidism, but is rarely encountered.

Lymphoedema

This is the accumulation of lymph in the dependent parts of the body due to either the congenital absence of lymphatics, or impaired lymphatic function resulting from recurrent infection, surgery, trauma or infiltration of lymph nodes or vessels with malignancy.

The swelling is said to be non-pitting, although pressure can cause slight pitting to occur.

Treatment

Treatment of the underlying cause is necessary, together with leg elevation and the use of compression stockings. Diuretics are of little benefit, as the fluid cannot reach the circulation to be excreted.

CASE
15

Cardiovascular disorders

CASE 16

The patient with high blood pressure

This is an extremely common station that can be used to test history taking, communication skills, clinical knowledge, therapeutics and pharmacology, but is mainly used to assess competence in the practical procedure of recording a blood pressure.

Hypertension

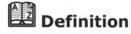 **Definition**

Because normal blood pressure tends to increase with age and is generally higher in men than in women, any definition must take these factors into account. A good definition is as follows: 'Hypertension is a blood pressure greater than 2 standard deviations above the mean of an age/sex-matched population'. As a rule of thumb the 'normal' systolic pressure is a value of approximately 100 mmHg + the chronological age of the patient in years (eg for a 20-year-old a normal systolic pressure is 120 mmHg, and for a 60-year-old it is 160 mmHg).

The normal value for diastolic pressure is approximately 80 mmHg. It, too, increases with age but the increase is much less. The diastolic pressure is extremely important, as it is the minimum pressure that is achieved within the systemic vascular tree and is therefore the minimum pressure that arteries must constantly withstand.

Excessively high pressure in arteries over a prolonged period of time leads to atheromatous change and arteriosclerosis, with all of the associated risks. Therefore it is vital to maintain both the systolic and diastolic pressure within an acceptable range, and in particular to ensure that the diastolic pressure remains below 90 mmHg.

As a general rule, blood pressure values that constitute hypertension are best considered in the following broad age bands:

- young adults (15–30 years)
- the middle-aged (30–55 years)
- the elderly (> 55 years).

CASE 16

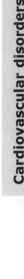

Hypertension	Systolic (mmHg)	Diastolic (mmHg)
Young adults	> 140	> 85
Middle-aged	> 160	> 90
Elderly	> 165	> 90

Values higher than these are potentially damaging to the vascular system, and the aim of therapy is to maintain the blood pressure below these levels.

? Causes

Hypertension can be classified as primary (idiopathic or essential) or secondary.

Treatment

A large number of drugs are available for the treatment of hypertension, and their mechanism of action varies. However, the class of drugs used and their mode of action can be easily remembered if one considers the factors that contribute to blood pressure, and the following formula:

$$BP = CO \times PR$$

where BP is blood pressure, CO is cardiac output (litres/minute) and PR is peripheral resistance.

Cardiac output is a function of heart rate and stroke volume:

$$CO = HR \times SV$$

where HR is heart rate and SV is stroke volume.

The blood pressure will decrease if drugs are used to reduce the following:

- heart rate (β-blockers)
- stroke volume (diuretics or β-blockers)
- peripheral resistance (calcium-channel blocking drugs, angiotensin-converting-enzyme (ACE) inhibitors, angiotension-II-receptor blocking drugs and nitrates.

A commonly used drug regime consists of introducing a single drug (eg diuretic) and, if the blood pressure is not well controlled by this, adding a second drug with a different mode of action (eg β-blocker or ACE inhibitor). If the blood pressure is still

CASE
16

not well controlled with the maximum tolerated dose of these drugs, a third class of drug is then added.

Essential hypertension

This accounts for more than 80% of cases of hypertension. There is no underlying disease process, but often there is a strong family history and other risk factors may be present. The underlying pathophysiology is increased vascular tone in the small arteries and arterioles, which causes a state of increased peripheral resistance.

Secondary hypertension

A variety of underlying disorders can result in the development of hypertension (see Table 4). In any patient newly diagnosed as hypertensive it is wise to investigate thoroughly to look for a remediable underlying cause.

Diagnosis

Clinical examination of the patient may reveal evidence of long-standing hypertension. The main abnormal clinical signs are as follows:

- elevation of blood pressure on repeated readings
- evidence of left ventricular hypertrophy – thrusting apex beat
- the presence of a fourth heart sound
- hypertensive retinopathy
- ECG changes consistent with left ventricular hypertrophy.

Measurement of blood pressure

This should be done after the patient has been allowed to relax for several minutes. Before taking the blood pressure it is wise to ask the patient if they have previously had their blood pressure checked. If they have not, explain the procedure and reassure them that although they may experience pressure in the area where the cuff is inflated and in their arm and hand, it is not painful, and tell them to inform you if they find it excessively uncomfortable, so that you can discontinue the procedure.

Ensure that the blood pressure recording apparatus is in good working order, and if you are using a sphygmomanometer that the reservoir of mercury is at approximately the same level as the patient's heart. Apply the cuff to the upper arm, ensuring that the patient's brachial artery is at the mid-point of the part which inflates. Apply the cuff neatly and firmly. Before you inflate the cuff, check the position of the pulse in the antecubital fossa and support the weight of the patient's

CASE
16

arm. With a palpating finger on the pulse, inflate the cuff until the pulse is no longer palpable and then continue inflating until the pressure rises by a further 20 mmHg. With your stethoscope in your ears gently put the diaphragm over the position of the brachial artery and slowly release the pressure in the cuff. The first sound that is heard corresponds to the systolic pressure. Note the pressure **exactly** (not to the nearest 5 or 10 mmHg) and continue to deflate the cuff while listening carefully. When the last Korotkoff sounds disappear, note the exact pressure. This corresponds to the diastolic pressure. Completely deflate the cuff and repeat the procedure twice more, but be sure to wait for 30 to 60 seconds between recordings. The blood pressure is taken as the mean value of the systolic and diastolic readings.

A number of factors can influence the readings that are obtained and the blood pressure may be elevated:

- if the patient has rushed into the consulting-room (their blood pressure may be elevated due to exercise)
- if the patient is anxious or nervous about having the test performed or about the result (white-coat hypertension)
- if the equipment is faulty
- if the cuff is too small for the size of the patient's arm – ensure that the cuff covers at least two-thirds of the circumference and one-third of the length of the arm
- if the patient has to hold their arm up unsupported
- if the cuff is repeatedly inflated and only partially deflated during a reading – always completely deflate the cuff and allow 30 to 60 seconds between recordings.

Hypertension is never diagnosed on the basis of a single blood pressure recording. If the pressure is found to be elevated, the whole procedure should be repeated on two more occasions after the patient has been relaxed for a period of 20 to 30 minutes.

CASE 16

Table 4 Classification of the causes of hypertension

Type	Cause
Essential (primary/idiopathic) (> 80% of cases)	Increased peripheral resistance (familial tendency)
Pregnancy	Pre-eclampsia
Vascular	Renal artery stenosis Coarctation of aorta
Endocrine/metabolic	Cushing's syndrome Conn's syndrome Phaeochromocytoma Acromegaly
Renal	All renal disorders that affect renal parenchyma
Other	Raised intracranial pressure Drugs (amphetamines, steroids, oral contraceptive pill) Alcohol

CASE 16

Cardiovascular disorders

CASE 17

Cardiac arrest

All doctors are expected to be able to identify and initiate management of a cardiac arrest. The ability to do this is commonly assessed at a must-pass station using a basic life support system or programmable mannequin.

Definition

Cardiac arrest is a condition in which there is no cardiac output sufficient to maintain life. The following three cardiac rhythm disorders are recognised causes of the condition:

1 asystolic arrest
2 ventricular tachycardia
3 ventricular fibrillation.

Clinical features

This is an acute medical emergency with sudden onset of loss of consciousness and hypotension. The patient will be collapsed, unresponsive and pale, with no pulse palpable and no recordable blood pressure. Unless basic life support measures are initiated within two minutes, the patient will suffer irreversible damage to the vital centres of the brain and any chance of recovery will be unlikely. It is vital that steps are taken quickly to assess the situation and initiate basic life support.

Signs of cardiac arrest include the following:

1 pale and pulseless
2 unconscious and unresponsive
3 no heart sounds audible.

CASE 17

Action to be taken

1 **Safety at the scene.** Ensure that there is no danger at the scene of the cardiac arrest. Put the patient in a supine position on a firm surface.

2 **Shout or send for help.**

3 **Airway.** Position the head in a tilted-back position, elevate the chin and look inside the mouth to ensure that there is a clear airway. Remove any material that could obstruct the airway (eg food debris, loose or false teeth, vomitus, etc).

4 **Respiration.** For 10 seconds look, listen and feel for evidence of respiration. Position your face over the patient's open mouth and watch for chest wall movement, listen for air movement and feel for the patient's breath on your cheek. Count out loud for 10 seconds – this makes bystanders aware that you are actually doing something active. If there are no signs of respiration, give two breaths by mouth-to-mouth ventilation.

5 **Circulation.** Check for evidence of a cardiac output – feel for a pulse at the carotid or femoral arteries. If none is palpable, give 15 chest compressions of cardiac massage.

6 **Life support.** Continue mouth-to-mouth ventilation and cardiac massage at a ratio of 2:15 until it is possible to establish what rhythm disturbance is present and a defibrillator arrives.

7 **Cardiac resuscitation.** When an ECG monitor or defibrillator arrives at the scene it is possible to establish which rhythm disturbance is responsible for the cardiac arrest. Monitoring pads should be applied to the chest – one in the right second interspace, mid-clavicular line, and one in the sixth interspace, anterior axiliary line. It is possible to re-establish sinus rhythm by direct current (DC) cardioversion if the arrhythmia is either ventricular tachycardia or ventricular fibrillation (see page 53). If asystole is present, DC cardioversion will have no effect.

Treatment of asystole

This cannot be reversed by DC cardioversion, and the only hope of re-establishing a cardiac rhythm is by injection of adrenaline (epinephrine) (10 ml of 1 in 1000 dilution) intravenously, and flushing into the circulation with 20 ml of 0.9% saline while continuing life support measures. Occasionally the effect of adrenaline is to stimulate a cardiac contraction, which may re-establish electrical activity.

**CASE
17**

Ventricular tachycardia/ventricular fibrillation

These forms of arrhythmia can potentially be converted to sinus rhythm using a DC defibrillator. The recommended sequence of events is as follows:

1 assess the rhythm to ascertain whether it is ventricular tachycardia (VT) or ventricular fibrillation (VF)

2 ensure that no one is in contact with the patient

3 defibrillate with DC energy of 200 joules

4 if the rhythm is still VT/VF, repeat DC cardioversion at an energy level of 200 joules

5 assess the rhythm. If it is sinus rhythm, give oxygen, support respiration, maintain blood pressure and monitor the cardiac rhythm

6 repeat step 4

7 if the rhythm is still VT/VF, defibrillate at an energy level of 360 joules

8 repeat step 4

9 if no cardiac output is established, continue cardiopulmonary resuscitation until further help arrives or it is clear that no recovery is possible.

Cardiovascular disorders

CASE
17

Respiratory disorders

CASE 18

The patient with shortness of breath

This is the second commonest clinical problem used in history-taking stations. It is used to assess the student's communications skills together with their ability to differentiate between the many clinical conditions that can present as dyspnoea.

Definition

Shortness of breath is the subjective sensation of increased respiratory effort.

? Causes

These can be classified either according to the rate of onset or in terms of the organ system that is affected.

Causes according to rate of onset

- Acute (within seconds to hours) – pneumothorax, pulmonary embolism, asthma, acute left ventricular failure, cardiac tamponade
- Paroxysmal – pulmonary oedema, asthma
- Weeks to months – cardiac failure, recurrent pulmonary emboli, pulmonary fibrosis, pleural effusion, lung cancer
- Years – chronic obstructive pulmonary disease (bronchitis/emphysema).

Causes according to organ system affected

Respiratory system

- Airflow obstruction – asthma, bronchitis, emphysema, tumour, pulmonary collapse of lobe or segment
- Reduced compliance – pulmonary fibrosis
- Impaired gas exchange – chest infection, consolidation, pulmonary oedema, pulmonary fibrosis, granulomatous disorders (eg sarcoidosis)
- Pleural disease – pleural effusion, pneumothorax.

CASE 18

Respiratory disorders

Cardiovascular disorders

1 Cardiac:

- left and/or right ventricular failure
- arrhythmias
- valvular disorders
- abnormal communications (septal defects)
- congenital abnormalities
- pericarditis
- pericardial effusion.

2 Vascular:

- pulmonary embolism.

Neuromuscular disorders

- Myasthenia gravis
- Guillain-Barré syndrome
- Polymyositis
- Polio.

Musculoskeletal disorders

- Ankylosing spondylitis
- Rheumatoid arthritis.

Other causes

- Pregnancy
- Obesity
- Anaemia.

Questioning should therefore be systematic and aimed at determining the rate of onset, the severity (as assessed by the patient's exercise tolerance), the rate of progression and associated symptoms. On the basis of these features it is usually possible to determine the most likely underlying cause.

Many of these features are dealt with as part of individual case histories in this book, while others should be revised in more comprehensive textbooks.

**CASE
18**

CASE 19

Asthma

This common respiratory problem can be used to assess the student's competence in history taking, physical examination, or ability to demonstrate and explain to patients the use of inhalers or peak flow meters.

Definition and classification

Asthma is an acute obstructive airways disease in which the FEV_1 is reduced to less than 80% of normal, and between attacks there is no evidence of any obstructive disorder.

Asthma can be classified as either extrinsic or intrinsic.

Extrinsic asthma

This usually has onset at an early age. It is more likely to occur in atopic individuals with a family history of asthma, hay fever or eczema, and is more common in males than in females.

A number of factors can precipitate acute attacks of shortness of breath. These can be remembered using the mnemonic **BASIC**:

- **B** – bronchial hyper-reactivity (eg to fumes, smoke, inhaled irritants)
- **A** – allergens
- **S** – stress
- **I** – infection
- **C** – cold temperature or lack of compliance with medication.

Intrinsic asthma

This condition usually has onset in adult life. There is no associated history of allergic disease, and it is more common in women than in men. There is a subcategory of this condition in which there is sensitivity to aspirin and non-steroidal anti-inflammatory drugs. These drugs inhibit arachidonic acid metabolism via the cyclo-oxygenase pathway. In certain individuals this leads to increased production of leukotrienes via the lipoxygenase pathway, which can trigger acute episodes of shortness of breath.

Clinical features

Patients describe episodes of sudden onset of shortness of breath with wheeze. In patients with extrinsic asthma this may be precipitated by the triggering factors mentioned above. There may be a cough that is productive of thick mucoid sputum.

Investigations

Investigations show a marked reduction in FEV_1 and a reduced partial pressure of oxygen in the arterial blood. Normally the partial pressure of carbon dioxide remains normal, but if it starts to rise this is a very sinister development and would indicate that the patient is starting to develop severe respiratory failure.

Treatment

Oxygen should be administered by inhalation at 100% concentration if necessary. Remove the triggering factor if present, and treat any underlying infection. Inhaled bronchodilators such as salbutamol and/or ipratropium bromide should be used. In severe cases, intravenous theophylline and intravenous hydrocortisone should be given, followed by a course of oral steroids.

If the patient develops severe respiratory failure with a rising carbon dioxide level, intermittent positive pressure ventilation or even ventilation in an intensive care unit should be considered.

Treatments aimed at preventing attacks include the identification and avoidance of triggering factors if present, the use of inhaled corticosteroids and regular monitoring of peak flow for any evidence of a reduction in FEV_1, which should be promptly treated with bronchodilators.

CASE
19

CASE 20

Chronic obstructive pulmonary disease (COPD)

This term is given to any lung disease in which there is a chronic obstruction to airflow that is not completely reversible. The two main causes are chronic bronchitis and pulmonary emphysema.

Chronic bronchitis

This is defined as the presence of cough productive of mucoid sputum for three or more consecutive months, for three or more consecutive years.

It is strongly associated with exposure to cigarette smoke and air pollution, and its incidence increases with age. Hereditary factors seem to play a role, possibly with regard to the amount and quality of mucous secretion in the lungs.

✎ Clinical features

Patients by definition have a chronic productive cough, with sputum production being more marked in the mornings. They have shortness of breath that is worse on exertion and which deteriorates progressively over a period of years. Acute exacerbations of symptoms can occur, and are often precipitated by cold temperature, exposure to air pollution, cigarette smoking or respiratory infection.

Pulmonary emphysema

This is a condition in which there is over-inflation of lung parenchyma with destruction of the normal architecture of the lung and the development of large air spaces. The change in lung architecture results in a reduced surface area for gaseous exchange. There is associated inflammation in the airways which, together with the over-distended alveoli, results in obstruction to airflow in the bronchioles.

✎ Clinical features

Patients with emphysema also develop shortness of breath, which becomes progressively worse over a number of years. There can be acute exacerbations due to intercurrent infection or exposure to irritants. Patients are more commonly plethoric in appearance due to the presence of secondary polycythaemia. Because of the increased respiratory rate that occurs in these patients, the partial pressure of carbon dioxide in the blood is reduced and they do not have the cyanotic appearance that is observed in patients with chronic bronchitis: they are 'pink puffers' rather than 'blue bloaters'.

Investigations

Chest X-ray often shows hyperinflated lungs with translucent lung fields, and bullae (large air spaces) may be present.

Patients may develop right ventricular failure secondary to the pulmonary hypertension, and are also prone to pneumothorax if a distended air space ruptures.

Treatment of COPD

Patients with these conditions should be strongly encouraged to stop smoking and to avoid exposure to environmental pollutants. The mainstay of therapy is the use of bronchodilator drugs by inhalation, together with inhaled steroids or systemic steroids to reduce the inflammatory reaction in the lungs. Any infective episodes should be treated promptly with appropriate antibiotics, and acute exacerbations will often require the use of inhaled oxygen. However, care must be taken not to prescribe oxygen at high concentrations in patients with chronic airways disease, as their respiratory drive is often dependent on hypoxia. If oxygen is inhaled at high concentration, the respiratory centre of the brain may fail to initiate regular respiratory efforts.

It is always wise to commence patients on 28% oxygen and to monitor arterial blood gases before increasing the concentration of oxygen.

CASE 20

CASE 21

Haemoptysis

This is an excellent history-taking topic, as it tests the student's ability to focus their questioning on several serious medical conditions and ask discriminating questions to determine the cause.

Definition

Haemoptysis is the expectoration of blood or bloodstained sputum.

Causes

These can be classified in order of prevalence as follows:

1 Respiratory causes:

- bronchogenic carcinoma
- bronchiectasis
- pulmonary embolism
- pneumonia
- pulmonary tuberculosis.

2 Haematological causes:

- warfarin (anticoagulation) excess
- haematological malignancies
- thrombocytopenia.

3 Cardiac causes:

- mitral stenosis.

4 Other causes:

- Goodpasture's syndrome.

CASE
21

It is useful to start by asking questions related to respiratory disease and, in particular, bronchogenic carcinoma (see Case 23), as this is the most common and most serious cause that must be ruled out. Do not forget to ask questions related to cigarette smoking (current and previous) and exposure to carcinogens during present or previous occupations (especially asbestos).

Weight loss and anorexia may occur in both bronchogenic cancer and tuberculosis, but the presence of drenching night sweats and a history of previous tuberculosis, exposure to someone with tuberculosis, or a patient from, or who has recently travelled to, a developing country should raise the possibility of tuberculosis. Sputum microscopy, cytology and culture are the best discriminating non-invasive tests to aid diagnosis.

Once you have ruled out respiratory causes, focus on the use of anticoagulants or other symptoms that might indicate a bleeding or clotting disorder (spontaneous bruising, bleeding of gums while cleaning teeth, nosebleeds, etc).

CASE
21

CASE 22

Chest infection

Chest infections are common clinical problems. They may occur as a primary disorder or secondary to some underlying condition such as other pathology in the lungs, or immunosuppressive or haematological disease. It is relatively rare to see patients during an acute episode of chest infection in clinical stations, although you may be asked to take a history from a simulated patient who has a chest infection. However, it is common to be assessed on interpretation of a chest X-ray in a radiology station with an X-ray showing an infective condition.

Definition

Pneumonia can be defined as inflammation of the substance of the lung. It may be caused by any type of micro-organism, but the commonest types of pneumonia which present to hospital are bacterial.

Clinical features

Pneumonia usually presents with an acute illness characterised by cough, purulent sputum and fever. The clinical findings are dependent on the stage of infection and to some extent on the type of organism that is causing the infection (see Table 5).

Table 5 Causes of chest infection

Organism	Frequency	Clinical circumstance
Streptococcal pneumonia	50%	Community-acquired
Mycoplasma pneumonia	5%	Community-acquired
Viral	5%	Community-acquired
Haemophilus influenzae	5%	Pre-existing COPD
Staphylococcus aureus	2%	Children, intravenous drug users, secondary to viral infection
Legionella pneumophila	2%	Institutional outbreaks
Pseudomonas	< 1%	Cystic fibrosis
No organism isolated	20%	

CASE 22

Chest infections can be broadly divided into two types, namely lobar pneumonia and bronchial pneumonia.

Lobar pneumonia

Lobar pneumonia is classically caused by *Streptococcus pneumoniae* infection, which accounts for approximately 50% of all community-acquired chest infections. It usually affects young adults, and more commonly occurs in the winter or early spring. It is spread by droplet infection, and most cases are sporadic.

Clinical features

The illness may be preceded by several days of flu-like symptoms with fever, which can rise to levels of 39–41°C. The patient then develops a cough productive of purulent sputum, and the illness may be complicated by pleurisy. On clinical examination there is reduced expansion on the affected side. As the disease progresses, the coarse crepitations which are initially present then disappear as the segment or lobe of the lung becomes consolidated. The classic signs of consolidation occur, with reduced or absent air entry, bronchial breath sounds, dullness to percussion, and increased vocal resonance and tactile vocal fremitus. If overlying pleural inflammation occurs, a pleural friction rub may be audible.

Investigations

Investigations show the presence of a raised white cell count, which is usually a polymorphonuclear increase. The chest X-ray classically shows features of a lobar pneumonia. Sputum culture often reveals the causative organism, and occasionally blood culture or urine culture may be positive.

Treatment

This usually consists of a penicillin antibiotic such as co-amoxiclav 1.3 g three times daily, but in patients who are allergic to penicillin, clarithromycin 500 mg twice daily can be used. Supportive measures such as the use of inhaled oxygen and adequate fluid balance are also required.

Bronchopneumonia

This condition more commonly affects young children, patients with chronic obstructive airways disease and the elderly. The most common causes are *Haemophilus influenzae* infection, *Streptococcus pneumoniae* and *Staphylococcus aureus*.

**CASE
22**

📝 Clinical features

The characteristic features are shortness of breath, cough and purulent sputum. On auscultation of the chest, the findings are of widespread or localised coarse crepitations that are heard in the affected areas.

Sputum culture is useful for identifying the organism and determining antibiotic sensitivities, but as a general guide the use of co-amoxiclav 1.2 g three times a day or clarithromycin 500 mg twice a day in patients who have penicillin allergy is usually effective. However, antibiotic treatment may need to be altered on the basis of sensitivity-testing results.

Respiratory disorders

CASE
22

Respiratory disorders

CASE 23

Bronchogenic carcinoma

Simulated patients are often used in the OSCE to give a history suggestive of an underlying bronchogenic neoplasm. It is unusual to encounter a real patient in this part of the examination. In the radiology station it is quite common to see a chest X-ray showing a lung tumour.

Definition and types

Bronchogenic carcinoma is a malignant transformation of tissue within the lung parenchyma. Five pathological cell types occur:

1 **Squamous-cell carcinoma** (40% of all lung tumours). This tumour arises from the surface epithelium of the bronchus and is strongly associated with cigarette smoking and exposure to asbestos. It spreads by direct extension to hilar nodes, and it metastasises late. The treatment is surgical resection.

2 **Large-cell lung tumour** (20%). This tumour is composed of large, poorly differentiated cells with abundant cytoplasm and variably sized nuclei. It often occurs in the periphery of the lung, is rapidly growing and metastasises early.

3 **Adenocarcinoma** (15%). This tumour shows an organised cellular pattern resembling bronchial glands. It usually occurs at the periphery of the lung, often in the sub-pleural region, and frequently arises around scar tissue. These tumours invade blood vessels and lymphatics at an early stage, and also spread to the pleura and mediastinal nodes. They commonly metastasise to bone and brain. There is no strong association with cigarette smoking, and they occur more commonly in women than in men.

4 **Small-cell lung tumour** (25%). This tumour arises from endocrine-type (APUD) cells and may secrete peptides. It is composed of small cells with dense hyperchromatic nuclei, and is sometimes known as 'oat cell' carcinoma. It is rapidly growing, metastasises early and spreads to lymph nodes and via the bloodstream. These tumours can be associated with endocrine abnormalities, as they may secrete active peptides such as adrenocorticotropic hormone (ACTH). The 5-year survival rate is less than 5%.

CASE 23

5 **Alveolar-cell carcinoma** (less than 2% of all lung tumours). These are rare tumours, and their appearance on X-ray is more like pulmonary fibrosis. They spread widely throughout the lung.

As a general rule, small-cell carcinoma shows a better response to chemotherapy than to surgical treatments, and non-small-cell carcinomas have a better prognosis with surgical resection. However, for all histological types the presence of metastases carries an extremely poor prognosis.

Clinical features

Characteristically these tumours do not present early. The symptoms that should suggest the possibility of an underlying bronchogenic tumour are as follows:

1 recurrent chest infections

2 failure of chest infections to resolve with appropriate antibiotic therapy

3 a change in the character of the cough

4 a reduction in the amount of sputum production by a smoker (due to obstruction to the drainage of a portion of the lung)

5 haemoptysis

6 hoarseness – when this occurs it may indicate paralysis of the left recurrent laryngeal nerve as it descends to the hilum before reflecting back to the larynx

7 weight loss associated with anorexia in a patient with respiratory symptoms.

On examination, the signs that might indicate the presence of a tumour are as follows:

1 reduced expansion of the affected lung or lobe of the lung

2 reduced air entry

3 a late-phase expiratory wheeze, due to air trapping in the affected lung

4 signs of collapse or consolidation distal to the tumour.

Respiratory disorders

CASE 23

Investigations

The initial investigations should be chest X-ray and sputum for cytology. If no tumour cells are obtained at cytology, a bronchoscopy with biopsy, bronchial washings or brushings may yield a tissue diagnosis. CT scanning is also helpful in patients with more distal tumours that cannot be seen at bronchoscopy, and for staging the tumour.

Treatment

The most effective treatments for the different types of lung tumour have been mentioned above, but treatment depends very much on the stage of the disease, the presence or absence of metastases and the general health and respiratory function of the patient.

Respiratory disorders

CASE
23

CASE 24

Pulmonary tuberculosis

There is still a considerable number of patients in the community with a past history of pulmonary tuberculosis, who may be used for physical examination of the chest showing abnormal clinical signs. It is rare to see a patient with acute pulmonary tuberculosis in the OSCE examination, although it is important for students to know the natural history of this condition.

Definition

Pulmonary tuberculosis is a pulmonary infection, caused by *Mycobacterium tuberculosis*, which often affects the apical region of a lung.

Infection usually begins as a patch or area of bronchopneumonia in the apical region of one lung, and the inflammatory response progresses to form caseous necrosis. Some of these foci may liquefy and discharge into the bronchial tree, resulting in cavity formation. Healing occurs with fibrosis, and cavities often persist with dormant virulent bacteria present.

Clinical features

In the acute phase, patients present with anorexia, fatigue, weight loss and drenching night sweats. They may also have a cough that is productive of mucoid or purulent sputum, and haemoptysis in small amounts is often present, particularly in advanced disease. If the area of inflammation in the lung extends to the pleural surface, pleuritic chest pain may be present.

On clinical examination the findings will depend on the stage of the condition. In the early stage of bronchopneumonia, reduced air entry and coarse crepitations may be heard, but as the disease progresses and cavitation occurs, signs of bronchial breathing and increased vocal resonance will develop. If there is significant fibrosis in the apex of the lung, the trachea may be pulled towards the affected side.

Investigations

Sputum samples may show the presence of a typical mycobacterial organism on direct microscopy. Sputum culture will again confirm the diagnosis, but it can take up to six weeks before a definite result is obtained. The chest X-ray often shows patchy inflammation in a superior or apical segment of the right or left lung, and cavity formation may be seen.

A full blood picture often shows a normochromic normocytic anaemia, and the white cell count may be normal or slightly elevated, with an increased absolute number of monocytes.

Patients who have what is termed 'open tuberculosis' (when organisms can be identified in the sputum) should be isolated and contacts should be screened for possible tuberculous infection.

Treatment

Pulmonary tuberculosis is treated in two phases:

1 an initial phase using triple drug therapy
2 a continuation phase during which two drugs are continued.

The initial phase of treatment is designed to reduce the bacterial population as rapidly as possible and prevent the emergence of drug-resistant bacteria. The drugs are best given as combination preparations unless there is some contraindication or there are signs of bacterial resistance or intolerance in the patient. Isoniazid, rifampicin and ethambutol combined with pyrazinamide are the drugs of choice. These drugs should be given for two months. Sputum cultures should be tested for drug sensitivity to ensure that the organism is sensitive.

During the continuation phase of treatment, isoniazid and rifampicin are given for four months.

The dosage of these drugs is dependent on the patient's body weight and must be determined on an individual basis.

CASE
24

Respiratory disorders

CASE 25

Pulmonary fibrosis

There are many patients with pulmonary fibrosis who are available to be used for clinical examinations, who can give an excellent history of chronic progressive pulmonary disease and have classic physical signs.

Definition

Pulmonary fibrosis is the replacement of normal lung architecture with fibrotic tissue, thus reducing the compliance of the lung and the surface area available for gaseous exchange.

? Causes

Any inflammatory process that affects the lung parenchyma can result in the deposition of fibrous tissue. However, a number of conditions are commonly associated with pulmonary fibrosis:

1 cryptogenic fibrosing alveolitis (idiopathic)

2 pulmonary tuberculosis

3 autoimmune disease – scleroderma (CREST), rheumatoid arthritis, systemic lupus erythematosus and chronic active hepatitis

4 there is an association with inflammatory bowel disease, especially ulcerative colitis

5 asbestosis

6 extrinsic allergic alveolitis.

Clinical features

Pulmonary fibrosis is most often the result of the idiopathic condition known as cryptogenic fibrosing alveolitis. This causes gradual and progressive shortness of breath with a cough productive of scanty quantities of mucoid sputum. The classic signs are reduced expansion, reduced air entry and medium or coarse crepitations (crackles) that are unchanged in character after coughing. Finger clubbing commonly

CASE 25

develops, and with the progressive deterioration in lung function, secondary polycythaemia and cyanosis often develop. Chest X-ray shows a 'ground glass' appearance in the mid- and lower zones.

Blood gas analysis demonstrates hypoxaemia and hypercapnia. Lung function tests reveal a restrictive lung defect with reduced transfer factor.

Treatment

This consists of supportive therapy with oxygen by inhalation and prompt treatment of any infective episodes to prevent further lung damage. Steroids and immunosuppressive drugs have been used, but with little evidence of any effect on the natural history of this progressive disease.

Extrinsic allergic alveolitis

This is a common cause of pulmonary fibrosis in farm workers, and occurs as a result of the inhalation of organic material. It is essential to consider from the occupational history whether or not the patient could have been exposed to such material. The clinical features are very similar to those of cryptogenic fibrosing alveolitis, although the area of lung affected more often involves the upper lobes. Other antigens involved in triggering the inflammatory process and fibrosis are listed in Table 6.

Table 6 Antigens responsible for triggering the inflammatory process and pulmonary fibrosis

Antigen	Source	Disease
Serum proteins	Bloom from pigeons	Pigeon fancier's lung
Micropolyspora faenii	Mouldy hay	Farmer's lung
Unknown	Cotton/linen dust	Byssinosis
Thermoactinomyces saccharii	Sugar cane	Bagassosis

If exposure to the offending antigen can be prevented, the disease process will be halted and the prognosis is excellent, although the damage that has already developed is irreversible.

CASE
25

CASE 26

Bronchiectasis

There are many patients in the community with this disorder who can be used for history-taking or clinical examination stations.

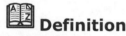 Definition

Bronchiectasis is a condition in which there is chronic infection within the lungs, which results in widening of the small bronchi, associated with increased mucus production.

The condition usually occurs after recurrent episodes of pneumonia, and is therefore more common in patients with cystic fibrosis or a primary immune deficiency disorder such as hypogammaglobulinaemia.

Recurrent inflammation of the lung tissue results in breakdown of the normal lung architecture and weakening of the bronchial walls. The increased traction on the walls from the surrounding tissues results in dilatation and the development of ectatic airways. The disease may be segmental in distribution, and more commonly affects the basal segments of the lungs, which can become chronically infected with organisms such as *Haemophilus influenzae*, pneumococci or staphylococcal organisms.

Clinical features

Patients have a cough productive of copious amounts of purulent sputum. They may have intermittent episodes of haemoptysis, and long-standing bronchiectasis can result in finger clubbing. On auscultation there are coarse crepitations in the affected area of the lung. Bronchiectasis can be complicated by recurrent infection, lung abscess formation, empyema, pneumothorax or amyloid disease.

Investigations

Chest X-ray shows increased lung markings in the affected region of the lung that have a 'honeycomb' appearance, sometimes associated with ring shadows containing fluid levels. CT scanning will confirm the presence of dilated airways containing mucus or infected secretions.

Treatment

Treatment consists of antibiotic therapy for acute exacerbations of infection, together with physiotherapy and postural drainage. Occasionally, localised areas of lung tissue can be surgically removed to prevent further recurrent infection. Any underlying immunodeficiency state should be corrected. For example, patients with hypogammaglobulinaemia should be given regular intravenous replacement immunoglobulin therapy.

CASE
26

CASE 27

Pneumothorax

This is commonly used as an X-ray station to test the student's knowledge of features used to diagnose the condition and identify the presence of a tension pneumothorax.

Definition

Pneumothorax is the presence of air between the parietal and visceral pleurae, usually associated with complete or partial collapse of the lung on the affected side.

Clinical features

It usually affects either healthy young adults or elderly patients with underlying lung disease, and the male:female ratio is 6:1. The commonest form of presentation is sudden onset of pleuritic-type chest pain and shortness of breath.

? Causes

- Spontaneous (primary/idiopathic)
- Rupture of emphysematous bulla
- Rupture of a cavitating lesion (eg tuberculosis, Wegener's granulomatosis)
- Gas-producing organism in a lung abscess (eg staphylococcal pneumonia)
- Trauma
- Underlying connective tissue disease (eg Marfan's syndrome)
- Positive-pressure ventilation
- Iatrogenic cause (eg after lung or pleural biopsy).

Clinical signs

- There is reduced expansion on the affected side
- The trachea is usually central, but if tension pneumothorax develops the trachea is pushed over to the other side

CASE 27

Respiratory disorders

- The chest is hyper-resonant on the affected side
- Breath sounds are diminished or absent.

If tension pneumothorax is present, the patient becomes increasingly short of breath and may develop cyanosis and hypotension, and the trachea is deviated to the opposite side of the neck.

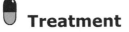

Investigations

Chest X-ray is usually confirmatory and shows hyperlucency on the affected side with no lung markings, and the edge of the collapsed lung is visible.

Treatment

Tension pneumothorax

This is an acute medical emergency and must be treated immediately by relieving the pressure on the affected side. This can be achieved by insertion of an open cannula or even making a stab wound and allowing the air under pressure to escape.

Non-tension pneumothorax

The choice of treatment is determined by the size of the pneumothorax:

- Small (< 25% of lung collapsed). This may not require any treatment. Monitor the patient and repeat chest X-rays. The air is often reabsorbed naturally.
- Moderate (25–40% of lung collapsed) (or if a small pneumothorax is causing respiratory distress). The air can be aspirated using a cannula and syringe via a three-way tap.
- Large (> 40% of lung collapsed) (or if a moderate pneumothorax is associated with respiratory distress). Insert an intercostal catheter and use an underwater seal drain to allow air to escape.

Complications

Around 50% of patients with primary spontaneous pneumothorax will have a recurrence on the same side. If two episodes occur, the risk of a third or fourth episode is greatly increased and surgical pleurectomy may be necessary.

CASE
27

CASE 28

Pleural effusion

Although this is not a common type of case encountered in the OSCE examination, there are many patients with pleural effusion available and willing to be used for examination purposes. The condition is most often used for clinical examination.

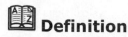 **Definition**

Pleural effusion is a collection of fluid in the pleural space, between the parietal and serosal layers of the pleura.

Classification

1 Transudates have a protein content of < 4 g/litre or a lactate dehydrogenase (LDH) concentration of < 200 mmol/litre

2 Exudates have a protein content of > 4 g/litre or an LDH concentration of > 200 mmol/litre.

? Causes

1 Transudates:

- cardiac failure
- hypoproteinaemia
- constrictive pericarditis
- Meigs' syndrome
- benign asbestos-related cause.

2 Exudates:

- haemothorax
- lobar pneumonia
- carcinoma (primary or secondary of pleura)

- pulmonary embolus
- tuberculosis
- empyema
- autoimmune disease (eg rheumatoid arthritis, systemic lupus erythematosus)
- mesothelioma.

Clinical features

The patient may have clinical features of the underlying cause together with increasing shortness of breath. The degree of dyspnoea is directly proportional to the amount of fluid in the pleural space. On examination, the classic physical signs are as follows:

1 The trachea is usually central, but with large effusions it may be deviated to the opposite site
2 Chest expansion is reduced on the side of the effusion
3 The chest is stony dull to percussion below the level of the fluid
4 Breath sounds are absent below the level of the fluid
5 At the air–fluid interface three additional signs are present:
   - bronchial breath sounds
   - aegophony – a bleating quality to the sounds of words
   - whispering pectoriloquy – an amplification of whispered words.

Investigations

The diagnosis is confirmed by chest X-ray, which shows the characteristic features.

In order to determine the nature and cause of the effusion, pleural aspiration is usually necessary. As large a sample as possible should be sent for biochemical analysis, bacteriological culture and microscopic examination, to look for evidence of malignant cells (cytology).

Treatment

Aspiration or drainage of the fluid relieves the symptom of shortness of breath. To prevent recurrence it is essential to establish and treat the underlying cause. For malignant effusions, once the fluid has been fully drained the instillation of cytotoxic drugs or irritants into the pleural space may prevent re-accumulation. If it does not, surgical excision of the pleura may be needed.

CASE
28

Gastrointestinal disorders

CASE 29

Dysphagia

This condition can be caused by a wide variety of disorders, and is used in a history-taking station to assess the student's ability to systematically rule out possible serious causes and ask the discriminating questions necessary to identify sinister pathology.

Definition

Dysphagia is difficulty with the act of swallowing, which may be due to pain or obstruction.

? Causes

Gastrointestinal causes

1 Oral causes – glossitis, stomatitis, aphthous or other ulceration, xerostomia, oral tumours

2 Pharyngeal causes – pharyngitis, pharyngeal pouch, neoplasm, post-cricoid web (Plummer-Vinson syndrome).

Oesophageal causes

Note: Common causes, accounting for more than 90% of cases, are shown in bold.

1 External compression – cervical or mediastinal nodes, thyroid enlargement, aortic aneurysm, carcinoma of bronchus, left atrial enlargement, pericardial effusion

2 Mechanical obstruction – **oesophagitis**, **stricture**, **carcinoma**, hiatus hernia, foreign body (including food bolus)

3 Motility disorders – **achalasia**, oesophageal spasm, systemic sclerosis

4 Gastric causes – carcinoma of the cardia

5 Neurological causes – myasthenia gravis, bulbar palsy, cranial nerve lesions (IX, X, XI or XII), motor neurone disease.

CASE 29

The following series of simple questions is used to help elucidate the underlying cause.

How long have you had difficulty with swallowing?

A history of less than one day would indicate a mechanical obstruction due to a foreign body or food bolus. Symptoms that have been present for a few weeks would be suggestive of oesophagitis, stricture or carcinoma. If symptoms have been present for months, external compression is the most likely underlying cause.

Was the onset acute or gradual?

Acute onset usually occurs with mechanical obstruction due to a foreign body or large food bolus, but can occur in patients with stricture, achalasia or carcinoma if they attempt to swallow a piece of food which is just too large to pass through the lumen of the oesophagus.

What is the rate of progression?

If the difficulty with swallowing is getting progressively worse, it may indicate the presence of an oesophageal tumour which is causing progressive narrowing of the lumen. With neurological conditions the difficulty with swallowing does not normally progress.

Is the problem worse with solids or liquids?

As a general rule, if the difficulty with swallowing is worse with solids, the underlying cause is more likely to be a mechanical problem. With neurological and motility disorders patients more often have problems with swallowing liquids, and often give a history of regurgitation of liquid through the nose.

With oesophageal carcinoma the initial swallowing difficulty is with large pieces of food, progressing to smaller and smaller pieces and then eventually difficulty with liquids.

What is the position where food lodges?

If food tends to lodge in the neck, the lesion is likely to lie in the pharynx or be due to compression by the cervical nodes, the thyroid or an aortic arch aneurysm. The lodging of food at the lower end of the sternum is more often due to oesophageal stricture, carcinoma or achalasia.

Gastrointestinal disorders

CASE 29

Are there any associated symptoms?

A history of preceding heartburn suggests a diagnosis of stricture, while the presence of symptoms such as muscle weakness or wasting or signs of a previous stroke suggests that the swallowing difficulty is due to a neurological cause. Pain or discomfort in the mouth suggests an oral cause, and features of thyroid dysfunction suggest external compression by the thyroid.

Have there been any changes in weight and appetite?

Although most patients with dysphagia lose weight, the benign causes are usually associated with a slow weight loss and an increase in appetite. In patients with oesophageal cancer there is a dramatic weight loss and anorexia.

The clinical features of the common and serious causes of dysphagia (ie oesophagitis, stricture, carcinoma and achalasia) should be revised and the discriminating questions that would differentiate between these disorders rehearsed (see Cases 30, 32 and 33).

Gastrointestinal disorders

CASE
29

CASE 30

Achalasia

This may be encountered in a history-taking station with a simulated patient complaining of difficulty with swallowing, regurgitation of food or weight loss. However, the condition is more commonly encountered at a radiology station with a barium swallow image.

📖 Definition

Achalasia is loss of oesophageal peristalsis and failure of the lower oesophageal sphincter to relax after swallowing. It is caused by degeneration of ganglion cells of the myenteric plexus of the oesophagus and the dorsal vagal nucleus of the medulla.

📝 Clinical features

In adult life the patient begins to develop difficulty with swallowing, which may be intermittent at first and relieved by drinking liquids to aid the swallowing process, or by changing position (eg standing up).

Later on, more persistent difficulty with swallowing develops and the patient starts to regurgitate large quantities of undigested food. Weight loss and nutritional deficiency states may become evident. If the patient develops aspiration of oesophageal contents into the trachea, recurrent aspiration pneumonia may occur.

Patients with long-standing achalasia are at increased risk of carcinoma of the oesophagus, perhaps due to the prolonged exposure of the epithelium to carcinogens in food and drink.

🔍 Investigations

Plain X-ray of the chest may show a dilated oesophagus in the superior mediastinum with the presence of a fluid level. The best radiological test is a barium swallow, which shows failure of normal peristaltic waves, failure of relaxation of the lower sphincter, and a dilated oesophagus with a smooth tapering to the oesophageal sphincter ('rat's tail sign').

CASE
30

Oesophageal manometry is an extremely useful diagnostic test which shows failure of the normal peristaltic waves and a significantly raised resting pressure of the lower oesophageal sphincter (LOS).

Treatment

Balloon dilatation of the LOS gives immediate and usually long-lasting relief of symptoms. If symptoms do recur, the procedure can be repeated. For patients who fail to improve, Heller's procedure (division of the muscular wall of the lower oesophagus) is usually effective, but symptoms of reflux can occur and there is the risk of post-operative perforation.

Gastrointestinal disorders

CASE
30

CASE 31

Hiatus hernia

This common condition, which occurs more often in women than in men, is a cause of retrosternal chest pain and is sometimes used in history-taking stations. The candidates are therefore required to differentiate between the symptoms of reflux oesophagitis and ischaemic heart disease.

Definition

There is herniation of a portion of the stomach through the oesophageal hiatus, often associated with reflux of acid and symptoms of oesophagitis.

? Causes

Any condition which increases the intra-abdominal pressure, such as obesity, pregnancy, the presence of ascites, coughing or tumour, can push the stomach up through the oesophageal sphincter. It may occur without any underlying precipitating cause in individuals who have a weakness at the hiatus where the oesophagus penetrates the diaphragm.

Clinical features

The vast majority of individuals with hiatus hernia are asymptomatic. However, heartburn is an early symptom of the condition and usually occurs after meals. It is sometimes associated with belching or hiccup, and is exacerbated by lying down or stooping. The pain is felt as a burning sensation retrosternally and may radiate up into the neck. Waterbrash is the sudden secretion of saliva into the mouth, which occurs as reflex salivation due to the presence of acid in the oesophagus.

If oesophagitis is caused by the action of peptic acid in the oesophagus, this can lead to stricture formation with eventual dysphagia (which is worse for solids, the patient experiencing food lodging at the lower end of the oesophagus).

Diagnosis is made on the basis of history, but can be confirmed by endoscopy. Barium swallow is an alternative method of diagnosis.

Treatment

Treatment is aimed at reducing the intra-abdominal pressure and treating any reflux oesophagitis and acidity. Patients are therefore advised to lose weight, to take frequent small meals rather than large ones, and to take their last meal of the day more than three hours before retiring to bed. Simple antacids can be used but, more commonly, proton-pump inhibitors are prescribed to abolish acid formation in the stomach and therefore totally relieve the symptoms of reflux oesophagitis. In some cases the patient requires surgical repair to reduce the hernia and tighten the sphincter, thus preventing herniation into the thoracic cavity.

Gastrointestinal disorders

CASE
31

Gastrointestinal disorders

CASE 32

Oesophageal stricture

This condition may appear in a history-taking station with the patient complaining of dysphagia, or in a radiology station when the student is shown a barium swallow X-ray.

Definition

There is a narrowing of the oesophagus which is usually benign, and which can result in dysphagia.

Causes

Oesophageal stricture most commonly occurs as a complication of hiatus hernia and reflux oesophagitis, and there is usually a preceding history of heartburn or retrosternal chest pain. The main causes are as follows:

- hiatus hernia with reflux oesophagitis
- systemic sclerosis (scleroderma)
- swallowing corrosives (bleach, acid, alkali, etc)
- drugs (non-steroidal anti-inflammatory drugs, potassium supplements)
- post-operative (after partial gastrectomy or oesophageal surgery)
- congenital stenosis.

Clinical features

Patients, who usually have a history of reflux, begin to experience difficulty swallowing, with food lodging at the lower end of the oesophagus. They may experience pain or discomfort to the extent that they sometimes induce vomiting in an effort to relieve their symptoms. When they vomit they regurgitate undigested food. Weight loss may occur, but is less marked than in patients with oesophageal cancer, and the appetite is usually preserved.

CASE 32

Investigations

Contrast radiology (barium swallow) shows narrowing of the lower end of the oesophagus with smooth edges, and no evidence of 'shouldering' (as in oesophageal cancer) or 'rat's tail sign' (as in achalasia). Endoscopy is also an excellent diagnostic test, together with biopsy or cytology to rule out malignancy.

Treatment

Oesophageal dilatation can be performed at the time of endoscopy using either rigid dilators or balloon dilatation. The underlying cause should be treated in an effort to prevent recurrence.

Gastrointestinal disorders

CASE
32

CASE 33

Oesophageal carcinoma

It would be most unusual to encounter a real patient with this condition in the exam. However, the topic often comes up as part of a history-taking station on dysphagia, or a radiology station where a barium swallow X-ray is shown and questions are asked about the nature, diagnosis and management of the condition.

Definition

Oesophageal carcinoma is a primary neoplastic tumour of the oesophagus (either squamous-cell carcinoma or adenocarcinoma, and rarely oat-cell type). Its incidence is 1 in 20,000 of the UK population. It is more common in men than in women, and there is an association with excess alcohol intake and underlying medical conditions such as Barrett's oesophagus, achalasia, chronic severe iron deficiency, pharyngeal pouch, hereditary tylosis and coeliac disease.

Clinical features

Patients usually describe progressive dysphagia, initially for solids and later for liquids. The dysphagia progresses over a period of a few months, and occasionally acute obstruction due to a large food bolus lodging at the site of obstruction can precipitate an acute event. Weight loss is rapid and profound, and patients also describe a loss of appetite. Iron deficiency anaemia may result from chronic blood loss and occasionally, if the tumour erodes into a blood vessel, haematemesis may occur. Chest pain usually only develops with local infiltration of the tumour.

On clinical examination the patient is cachectic, they may have signs of anaemia, and cervical lymph nodes may be present. An irregular hepatomegaly may develop if there is secondary spread.

Investigations

Investigations that are diagnostic for this condition are endoscopy with biopsy or barium swallow.

💊 Treatment

Radical surgery offers the only chance of prolonged survival with this condition. Chemotherapy is sometimes used for adenocarcinoma but, overall, the 5-year survival rate is less than 10%.

CASE
33

Gastrointestinal disorders

CASE 34

The patient with weight loss

This provides an excellent history-taking station and is useful to assess students' ability to ask the discriminating questions that will identify an organic or psychiatric cause of this symptom.

📖 Definition

There is a reduction in total body weight.

❓ Causes

Gastrointestinal causes

- Dietary deficiency
- Any cause of dysphagia
- Gastric carcinoma
- Gastric ulceration
- Coeliac disease
- Crohn's disease
- Other causes of malabsorption.

Endocrine/metabolic causes

- Hyperthyroidism
- Malignancy of any organ or tissue
- Psychiatric causes (anorexia nervosa, bulimia, depression).

CASE 34

Other causes

- Infection, especially tuberculosis
- Chronic inflammatory disease (eg rheumatoid arthritis).

Clinical features

It is important to determine three main factors at the outset:

1 amount of weight loss – how many pounds, stones or kilograms of body weight have been lost

2 duration – over what period of time the weight loss has occurred

3 dietary intake and appetite – how the appetite has changed in association with weight loss.

Patients with most forms of gastrointestinal disease, especially malabsorption, and also those with hyperthyroidism, have weight loss associated with an increased appetite. Patients with underlying malignancy, infection or chronic inflammatory disease have weight loss associated with anorexia. Patients with gastric ulceration have weight loss and feel hungry, but are afraid to eat because they associate food intake with an exacerbation of the pain associated with acid secretion after meals.

As a general rule, rapid and profound weight loss with loss of appetite indicates serious underlying disease. A small amount of weight loss over a prolonged time period with normal appetite is usually less serious.

Patients with depression lose weight as a result of dietary neglect and loss of interest in food. Their weight loss is not usually excessive, and their mental state is diagnostic.

Patients with anorexia nervosa or bulimia are usually female (the female:male ratio is approximately 400:1). They have a distorted body image, and although they look wasted and frail they feel that they are overweight. Often they abuse laxatives and/or induce vomiting, which may result in electrolyte disturbances such as hypokalaemia.

Patients with anorexia frequently lose more than 25% of their ideal body weight, and have amenorrhoea, hair loss and lanugo.

Gastrointestinal disorders

CASE
34

CASE 35

Coeliac disease

This condition is the commonest cause of malabsorption in the UK, and could be encountered in a history-taking station with a patient who has symptoms of weight loss. It is occasionally used in data interpretation stations with biochemical features of malabsorption together with the usual antibody abnormalities associated with this disorder.

Definition

Coeliac disease is a gluten-sensitive enteropathy which results in a reduction in the total surface area of the small bowel that is available for absorption, often leading to features of malabsorption.

Clinical features

Coeliac disease affects approximately 1 in 3000 of the UK population. It can occur in any age group, but most commonly presents in children or young adults. Worldwide there is geographical variation in the incidence of the disease, which is more common in Russia and Ireland (in Galway the prevalence is 1 in 300) and very rare in Africa and Asia. It is a hypersensitivity reaction to the gliadin component of gluten, which is a water-soluble protein fraction of cereal grains (wheat, barley, rye and oats). When gliadin comes into contact with the small bowel, an intense inflammatory reaction develops which leads to subtotal or total villous atrophy and a dramatic reduction in the surface area of mucosa available for absorption. In children, failure to thrive (ie gain body weight or increase in height) is the usual reason for referral to specialist clinics. In adults, symptoms of deficiency states, especially iron deficiency anaemia, are the most common presentation. However, weight loss with a ravenous appetite, frequent bowel motions or steatorrhoea may be present.

Dermatitis herpetiformis

This is a vesicular, intensely itchy skin rash, which most commonly occurs over the extensor aspect of the limbs, especially around the elbows and knees, but may also be found on the buttocks and face. The itch is relieved by the patient scratching the skin and bursting the tiny vesicles. This rash is strongly associated with coeliac

CASE
35

disease, and is a cutaneous manifestation of gluten sensitivity. Deposition of immunoglobulin A occurs in the rete pegs of the dermis and can be visualised on skin biopsy using fluorescent stains and microscopy.

If left untreated, coeliac disease is associated with an increased risk of small bowel lymphoma.

Investigations

The full blood picture often shows anaemia due to iron deficiency and/or folate deficiency. Biochemical assays may show features of hypoproteinaemia and calcium and phosphate deficiency.

A glucose tolerance test gives a flat response consistent with malabsorption.

The presence of anti-endomysial antibodies and tissue transglutaminase is highly specific for this disorder. Duodenal or jejunal biopsy with microscopy usually shows subtotal or total villous atrophy, with inflammatory cells in the intra-epithelial spaces and a chronic inflammatory reaction in the lamina propria of the bowel wall.

Treatment

The total and lifelong avoidance of all food products containing wheat, barley, rye or oat flour is the best form of treatment. Expert dietary advice is essential, and plenty of support and encouragement is needed as this diet places a major restriction on the types of foods that the patient can enjoy.

Failure to respond to this regime is usually the result of the patient accidentally ingesting gluten or not complying fully with the elimination diet. Rarely, despite full compliance, malabsorption does persist, with features of an inflammatory enteropathy as seen on biopsy. These patients may require steroid or immunosuppressive drug therapy, but this should be managed at a specialist clinic as they are at risk of developing small bowel lymphomas and will require detailed investigation and regular follow-up.

Gastrointestinal disorders

CASE
35

CASE 36

Gastric carcinoma

It is unusual to encounter a real patient with gastric carcinoma in an OSCE examination unless they have had a resection. More commonly, a simulated patient will describe the typical features of this condition.

Definition

Gastric carcinoma is a malignant transformation of the gastric mucosa. It is more common in men than in women, occasionally occurring with a positive family history, and is more common in patients with blood group A than in those with other blood groups.

Clinical features

This condition is not usually associated with pain in the early stages. The most common presenting symptoms are of anorexia and weight loss, which can be profound. Patients often describe a feeling of fullness after eating a small quantity of food. Classically they describe sitting down for a meal but after two or three mouthfuls of food feeling that they cannot eat any more. Some patients present with symptoms of iron deficiency anaemia, and occasionally ulceration occurs on the tumour, causing dyspepsia.

On examination, the patient usually appears wasted with evidence of significant weight loss and muscle wasting. If the gastric tumour is causing pyloric outlet obstruction, visible peristalsis may be seen in the abdomen. A mass may be palpable in the upper abdomen, and if there is spread to the liver, hepatomegaly can be found. The presence of an irregular liver surface with umbilication of the nodules is said to be a classic finding.

The diagnosis is based on history and endoscopy with biopsy.

Treatment

The prognosis of this condition is extremely poor, and the only hope of effecting a cure is by partial or total gastrectomy. The 5-year survival rate is less than 2%.

CASE 36

CASE 37

Pancreatic carcinoma

It is extremely unlikely that a patient with pancreatic cancer would be encountered in an OSCE examination. However, students are expected to have a good knowledge of this serious disorder, which could be a cause of weight loss, anorexia and obstructive jaundice. A simulated patient who describes these symptoms is often used at a history-taking station.

Definition

Pancreatic carcinoma is a malignant tumour that arises from pancreatic tissue (most often adenocarcinoma which develops from ductal epithelium).

Clinical features

Pancreatic cancer may occur at any age, but is rare in those under the age of 40 and most common in people over the age of 60. The presentation varies depending on the site of the tumour.

Tumour of the head of pancreas

This usually presents with features of obstructive jaundice, which is commonly painless in the early stages. The patient develops weight loss and anorexia. Examination shows the presence of jaundice, and the liver may be enlarged and have an irregular surface if secondary deposits are present. Because of the obstruction to the biliary system, the gallbladder can become distended and may be palpable.

Note: In a patient with painless jaundice and a palpable gallbladder, always suspect carcinoma of the pancreas and remember Courvoisier's law. This states that in a jaundiced patient, a distended palpable gallbladder is unlikely to be due to stones (this is because if stones had been present in the gallbladder, the wall would have become thickened and fibrosed and would therefore be less likely to distend).

Tumour of the body or tail of pancreas

These tumours do not cause jaundice unless there is spread to the liver or to nodes in the porta hepatis. Most often they present with anorexia and profound weight loss,

CASE 37

and little is found on clinical examination. Pain develops at a relatively early stage, is in a central abdominal location and is classically relieved by leaning forward.

Investigations

Serological tests are not usually helpful, although certain tumour-specific antigens, such as CA19-9 and carcinoembryonic antigen (CEA), may be elevated in some patients.

Diagnosis requires either ultrasound scanning, CT or magnetic resonance imaging (MRI) scanning of the abdomen, or endoscopic retrograde cholangiopancreatography (ERCP). These techniques will only identify the presence of a mass or tumour.

If liver deposits are present, biopsy will allow histological identification. Fine-needle aspiration of the pancreatic tumour can result in fistula formation and has a very high false-negative rate for diagnosis.

Treatment

This condition has an extremely poor prognosis (85% of patients with pancreatic cancer die within one year of diagnosis). It is usually managed by treatment of the symptoms and palliative therapy. Obstructive jaundice should be relieved either by placing stents endoscopically or by surgical bypass of the obstruction. Chemotherapy and radiotherapy can be used to reduce the size of the primary tumour, but are of little benefit in improving survival. Surgery is used if there is limited disease with no evidence of spread.

CASE
37

CASE 38

Pancreatic insufficiency

This condition must be considered in a history-taking station where the patient has features of abdominal pain, weight loss and other symptoms suggestive of malabsorption.

Definition

Pancreatic insufficiency is failure of the pancreas to perform its exocrine function, usually as a result of chronic or repeated attacks of acute inflammation (pancreatitis).

? Causes

Any condition that increases the risk of infection in the pancreatic gland, or exposure to infectious agents or toxins which cause pancreatic inflammation, can lead to fibrosis and inability of the gland to perform its usual exocrine function.

By far the commonest cause is excessive alcohol consumption. The major causes of pancreatic insufficiency are as follows:

- excessive alcohol consumption
- gallstones
- chronic infection
- hyperlipidaemia
- fibrocystic disease
- idiopathic causes.

Patients give a history of acute attacks of upper abdominal pain, which is usually very severe and associated with vomiting. The pain is epigastric, radiates through to the back and is only partially relieved by leaning forward. After a number of bouts of acute pancreatitis, weight loss and steatorrhoea develop as the digestion of protein and fat is markedly impaired.

Loss of the endocrine function can occur, resulting in diabetes mellitus, but usually islet cell function is preserved until very late in the disease.

Gastrointestinal disorders

CASE
38

Few specific physical signs are observed, but features of nutritional deficiency and general features of malabsorption are present.

Investigations

During acute bouts of abdominal pain there is a significant rise in serum amylase levels, but in chronic disease the levels of this enzyme are normal. X-ray of the abdomen may show pancreatic calcification.

Pancreatic function can be assessed using the para-aminobenzoic acid (PABA) excretion test. This is performed by giving the patient a meal containing PABA which is attached to a protein. The patient must perform a 24-hour collection of urine after the test meal has been given. If there is sufficient pancreatic function to digest the protein component of the test meal, free PABA is excreted in the urine. The quantity of PABA excreted in the urine is directly proportional to the functional capacity of the exocrine pancreatic gland.

Treatment

1 Treat any underlying cause (ie encourage the patient to abstain from alcohol, remove gallstones, etc)

2 Pancreatic enzyme supplements taken with meals can prevent further weight loss and nutritional deficiency

3 Correct any electrolyte or nutritional deficiency states that are present

4 If endocrine function is deficient, insulin therapy may be required.

CASE
38

CASE 39

Crohn's disease

This condition may be encountered at a radiology station as a barium X-ray, or at a history-taking station with the patient complaining of symptoms of abdominal pain and altered bowel habit.

Definition

Crohn's disease is an inflammatory disease of unknown aetiology which can affect any part of the gastrointestinal tract from the mouth to the anus, but which most often causes symptoms due to small intestinal involvement.

Clinical features

This condition can affect people of all ages, but most often affects young adults, with onset in the 15–30 years age group. It is more common in women than in men.

Patients develop episodic bouts of crampy abdominal pain that may be associated with diarrhoea and weight loss. The pattern of symptoms varies depending on the site and extent of the inflammatory process. If the disease is mainly in the small intestine, features of malabsorption such as weight loss, steatorrhoea and nutritional deficiency predominate. If the rectum or large bowel is mainly involved, rectal bleeding or bloody diarrhoea is the predominant feature.

On examination of the abdomen an inflammatory mass may be palpable. This is commonly felt in the right iliac fossa, since there is frequently involvement of the terminal ileum. When this occurs it can be mistaken for an appendix abscess. A number of extra-intestinal manifestations of Crohn's disease may occur (see Table 7).

The non-caseating granulomatous inflammation which affects the full thickness of the intestinal wall can result in a variety of complications:

1 impaired absorption – with the development of malabsorption and nutritional deficiency states

2 stricture formation – this can result in intestinal obstruction

3 perforation – small perforations of the bowel can occur. These are usually contained locally, but can cause inflammatory masses or intraperitoneal abscesses

CASE 39

4 fistula formation – abnormal communications develop between inflamed loops of bowel, or between the bowel and the skin surface, bladder or female genital tract

5 anal fissures and fistulae – if the anus is involved, as it commonly is, the patient may develop painful fissures or discharging fistulae around the anal margins or on the buttocks.

Table 7 Extra-intestinal manifestations of inflammatory bowel disease

Constitutional manifestations	Weight loss
	Malaise
	Fever
Skin	Erythema nodosum
Joints	Asymmetrical large-joint arthropathy
	Sacroiliitis
	Ankylosing spondylitis
Ocular manifestations	Uveitis
	Episcleritis
Hepatic manifestations	Fatty infiltration
	Chronic active hepatitis
	Sclerosing cholangitis
Renal manifestations	Amyloid

Investigations

The full blood picture may show evidence of iron deficiency anaemia due to malabsorption. Markers of acute inflammation (erythrocyte sedimentation rate and C-reactive protein) are elevated, particularly during episodes of disease activity. Biochemical assays may show features of malabsorption (low albumin levels, calcium, vitamin B_{12} or folate deficiency).

Imaging of the bowel

If the disease is affecting the anus, rectum or sigmoid colon, proctoscopy or sigmoidoscopy allows direct visualisation and biopsy, which can confirm the diagnosis. For small bowel disease, barium studies are necessary. These may show bowel wall thickening, with narrowing of the lumen (string sign of Kantor), fistula formation, abnormal communication between loops of bowel, ulceration of the bowel mucosa

CASE
39

with 'collar-stud' or 'rose-thorn' ulcers, or a 'cobblestone' appearance of the mucosal surface.

💊 Treatment

The main aims of treatment are as follows:

- to reduce the inflammatory reaction in the bowel
- to correct any nutritional deficiency that has developed
- to treat any complications that have arisen.

The nature of the illness should be fully explained to the patient and their close relatives. Expert dietary advice should be given, and supplements prescribed to correct nutritional deficiencies.

Anti-diarrhoeal medication can be used to reduce the frequency of bowel movements. Specific anti-inflammatory drugs that can be used include corticosteroids, which can be given in the form of topical enemas or suppositories for anal, rectal or sigmoid colon disease.

For inflammation of the small bowel, which is not amenable to topical therapy, systemic therapy is used in the form of prednisolone. The dose prescribed will vary depending on the age of the patient and the severity of the disease.

Mesalazine (5-aminosalicylic acid) is a drug that allows the delivery of the anti-inflammatory salicylate to the lower parts of the gastrointestinal tract, and it can be used for both small and large bowel Crohn's disease. It is mainly used to prevent relapse, but it can be prescribed to reduce an acute flare-up of the disease.

The immunosuppressive drug azathioprine is prescribed as a steroid-sparing agent and is useful during severe episodes of disease activity.

Anticytokine drugs

Monoclonal antibodies that inhibit the interleukin cytokines or tumour necrosis factor are currently being used to good effect in patients with inflammatory bowel disease. These agents modulate the immunological reaction that causes the inflammatory damage, and they can suppress acute attacks. The use of these drugs may carry the risk of increased susceptibility to other infections, and their prolonged or repeated use may increase the risk of subsequent malignancies by suppressing the body's natural tumour surveillance mechanism.

Gastrointestinal disorders

CASE
39

CASE 40

Ulcerative colitis

This condition could be encountered at a history-taking station where the patient has symptoms of altered bowel habit, or at a radiology station where the student is shown a barium enema.

Definition

Ulcerative colitis is an idiopathic chronic inflammatory disorder of the gastrointestinal tract that usually affects the large bowel.

Clinical features

This condition can occur at any age, but most often has onset in the 20–40 years age group. It is more common in women than in men. Patients experience episodes of abdominal pain, increased bowel frequency (which may be associated with diarrhoea) and the passage of blood and mucus in the stools. The severity and duration of symptoms vary, and between attacks the patient may be completely asymptomatic.

During severe or prolonged attacks there may be constitutional symptoms of malaise, fever, anorexia and weight loss, and a number of extra-intestinal manifestations may complicate the illness. These are identical to those associated with Crohn's disease (see Table 7, page 104), but, in addition, the skin condition pyoderma gangreosum can occur.

Investigations

A full blood picture may show anaemia as a result of blood loss (iron deficiency) and a raised white cell count. The erythrocyte sedimentation rate and C-reactive protein level are elevated during episodes of disease activity.

Examination of bowel motion shows the presence of blood and inflammatory cells but no evidence of infective agents.

Gastrointestinal disorders

Radiology

Plain X-ray of the abdomen is essential in patients with an acute flare-up, as the life-threatening condition of toxic megacolon can develop. If this is present, the X-ray will show marked dilatation of the large bowel, and free air may be seen in the peritoneal cavity under the right hemidiaphragm, which would indicate perforation of the bowel.

In less acute disease, barium enema shows a featureless colon (loss of haustrations) with areas of superficial ulceration of the mucosa.

Direct visualisation

Sigmoidoscopy or colonoscopy provides direct visualisation of the colon and, together with biopsy, can be used to confirm the diagnosis histologically and monitor the response to treatment. However, with these procedures there is a risk of causing perforation, especially in patients with a severe inflammatory episode.

Treatment

Supportive treatment

The nature of the condition should be fully explained to the patient and their relatives.

Medication to reduce the frequency and severity of diarrhoea can be prescribed and any anaemia and electrolyte or nutritional deficiency corrected. Patients with profound blood loss may require transfusion.

The patient should be informed that an acute flare-up may be triggered by factors such as emotional stress, intercurrent infection, non-steroidal anti-inflammatory drugs, antibiotic treatment, food poisoning, gastrointestinal infection or any dietary indiscretion which causes episodes of diarrhoea.

Specific therapy

1 **Medical therapy.** Drugs that suppress the inflammatory reaction are the mainstay of treatment of this condition. These include the following:
   - corticosteroids used topically (by enema or suppository), orally or intravenously, depending on the severity of attacks
   - 5-aminosalicylic acid – an oral anti-inflammatory salicylate that is used mainly to prevent recurrence or relapses. Patients on long-term treatment with this type of preparation have a reduced annual relapse rate of 25%, compared with 75% for untreated patients.

Gastrointestinal disorders

CASE
40

- immunosuppressive drugs (eg azathioprine) – these drugs are used either to reduce the relapse rate or during acute attacks for their corticosteroid-sparing dosage effect.

2 **Surgical treatment.** Patients who fail to respond to medical treatment or who develop perforation or toxic megacolon often require total colectomy.

Patients with a history of ulcerative colitis for more than 15 years have an increased relative risk of developing carcinoma of the colon. Regular outpatient follow-up and annual colonoscopy are advised for these individuals.

Gastrointestinal disorders

CASE
40

CASE 41

Peptic ulceration

Peptic ulceration may be encountered at a history-taking station with a simulated patient complaining of upper abdominal pain and haematemesis. The student would be expected to ask the relevant questions for diagnosing a peptic ulcer, and should be able to differentiate between a gastric ulcer and a duodenal ulcer.

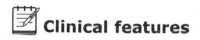

Definition

Peptic ulcer is a break in the mucosa close to the acid-secreting areas of the gastrointestinal tract. It usually occurs in the stomach or proximal duodenum, but may rarely affect the oesophagus, jejunum or a Meckel's diverticulum if it contains gastric acid-secreting mucosa.

Clinical features

Gastric ulceration

This condition most commonly affects older people, and is more frequently found in the socially deprived than in those of social class I or II. It is associated with *Helicobacter pylori* infection in 70% of cases, and can also be caused by ingestion of aspirin or non-steroidal anti-inflammatory drugs.

The patient complains of epigastric pain which may radiate through to the back. The pain is more severe after food, and is relieved by not eating. Consequently, although they feel hungry, the patient avoids food because they know that it will cause pain, and as a result they are usually thin.

If the ulcer erodes a blood vessel, bleeding into the stomach can occur and the patient may develop haematemesis and/or melaena (the passage of black, tarry, offensive-smelling stools). Other causes of haematemesis are shown in Table 8.

CASE 41

Table 8 Causes of haematemesis

Location	Cause
Oesophagus	Oesophagitis
	Mallory-Weiss tear
	Varices
	Carcinoma
Stomach	Gastric ulcer
	Acute gastritis
	Drugs (aspirin, non-steroidal anti-inflammatory drugs)
	Alcoholic gastritis
	Telangiectasia
	Haemorrhagic disorder
Duodenum	Duodenal ulcer
	Duodenitis
	Aortoduodenal fistula
	Pancreatic tumour infiltration
Other	Blood swallowed from nose, throat or respiratory tract

If the ulcer erodes through the full thickness of the stomach wall, perforation of the stomach may cause life-threatening peritonitis. If ulceration and scarring occur in the pyloric region of the stomach, outlet obstruction may result, causing severe abdominal pain and projectile vomiting, visible peristalsis in the epigastrium and a positive gastric splash test.

Duodenal ulceration

This also causes severe sharp epigastric pain which can radiate through to the back and may be associated with haematemesis and melaena. However, this pain is relieved by food or by taking antacids (both dilute or neutralise the acidity of fluid reaching the area of ulceration). The pain is worse when the patient is hungry, and therefore occurs before meals and classically awakens the patient from sleep in the early hours of the morning. Because food relieves the pain, these patients are often overweight.

Severe blood loss and perforation are both serious, life-threatening medical emergencies which must be identified and treated quickly.

CASE
41

Investigations

Although both types of ulceration can be identified on barium X-ray, the best diagnostic test is endoscopic examination of the stomach and duodenum. This allows direct visualisation of the ulcer. Any bleeding points can be identified and dealt with by cryotherapy, injection or laser coagulation. Biopsies can be taken to rule out gastric malignancy, and to look for evidence of *Helicobacter pylori*. This is a spiral, urease-containing bacterium that is found in 90% of patients with duodenal ulceration and 70% of patients with gastric ulcers. It plays a role in the inflammatory reaction in the stomach that leads to mucosal damage.

Treatment

The aims of treatment are to heal the ulceration and prevent recurrence. There are two main strategies:

1 *Helicobacter pylori* **eradication.** If this organism is identified, antibiotic therapy is used to kill the organism. A combination of amoxicillin, metronidazole and a proton-pump inhibitor is used, provided that the patient has no history of penicillin allergy (if they do, clarithromycin is substituted for the amoxicillin).

2 **Gastric acid suppression.** A variety of drugs are available which can inhibit the production or secretion of gastric acid. They include histamine H_2-receptor-blocking drugs (eg cimetidine, ranitidine) and proton-pump inhibitors (eg omeprazole, lansoprazole), which block the parietal cell H^+/K^+-ATPase proton pump and inhibit the release of H^+ ions into the stomach.

The potent action of these drugs has revolutionised the management of peptic ulcer disease, and it is seldom necessary for patients to undergo surgery to treat these disorders except in the event of severe haemorrhage which cannot be controlled by endoscopic methods, or if perforation occurs. When discussing the treatment of these disorders, it is important to be familiar with the management of acute blood loss, when and how to give blood transfusions, and how to recognise and manage acute peritonitis.

Gastrointestinal disorders

CASE
41

Gastrointestinal disorders

CASE 42

Chronic liver failure

This is an extremely common clinical examination station where the student will be asked to examine a patient who has multiple stigmata of chronic liver failure and/or to palpate the abdomen of a patient with liver enlargement or splenomegaly with or without ascites.

Definition

Chronic liver failure occurs as a result of irreparable damage to the liver, usually associated with liver cirrhosis.

Causes

Any recurrent or chronic disorder that causes liver cell damage may eventually lead to liver cell necrosis, deposition of fibrous tissue and nodular regeneration, which are the three hallmarks of liver cirrhosis. The major causes of chronic liver failure are as follows:

- alcoholic hepatitis
- viral hepatitis (especially chronic infection with hepatitis A or C)
- autoimmune disease (chronic active hepatitis)
- metabolic liver disease (Wilson's disease, haemochromatosis)
- ascending infection (ascending cholangitis).

Clinical features

The clinical features are numerous, and all of them occur as a direct result of failure of hepatic cell function. The major features are listed in Table 9.

CASE
42

Table 9 Clinical signs of chronic liver disease

Location	Signs
Skin	Jaundice
	'Paper-money' skin
	(thin skin with little supporting connective tissue)
	Excoriations
	Spider naevi
	Petechiae, purpura or ecchymoses
Hands	Palmar erythema
	Leuconychia
	Finger clubbing
	Flapping tremor
Abdomen	Hepatomegaly
	Splenomegaly
	Ascites (shifting dullness/fluid thrill)
	Caput medusae
Central nervous system	Confusion
	Constructional apraxia
Other	Gynaecomastia
	Testicular atrophy
	Loss of male secondary sexual characteristics
	Foetor hepaticus
	Peripheral oedema

The accumulation of ascites in the peritoneal cavity occurs as a result of the following:

- increased hydrostatic pressure in the blood vessels that drain into the portal vein
- reduced oncotic pressure of the blood due to hypoalbuminaemia
- elevation of aldosterone levels due to failure of the breakdown of aldosterone that normally occurs in the liver
- increased levels of other mineralocorticoids that would normally be metabolised by hepatocytes.

Gastrointestinal disorders

CASE
42

Complications

Patients with chronic liver failure can develop a number of potentially serious complications:

1 **Hepatic encephalopathy.** Because of the failure to convert nitrogenous waste products into urea, increasing levels of ammonia accumulate in the blood as a result of a large protein intake, intestinal haemorrhage, infection or trauma. If the ammonia levels rise excessively, this can cause suppression of higher cerebral functions and lead to an altered level of consciousness.

2 **Haemorrhage.** Failure of the liver to produce vitamin K-dependent clotting factors results in a tendency to bleed easily, and this can lead to spontaneous bleeding or major haemorrhage from internal organs.

3 **Oesophageal varices.** The increased resistance to blood flow through a cirrhotic liver causes increased hydrostatic pressure in the vessels that drain into the portal vein. At sites where the portal and systemic veins anastamose (eg the lower region of the oesophagus) varicosities can develop. These may spontaneously rupture, causing haematemesis which, because of the associated defect in coagulation, can be life-threatening and extremely difficult to control.

4 **Infection.** Chronic liver failure is a cause of secondary immunodeficiency, and patients are at increased risk of infection. They are particularly susceptible to peritonitis due to the presence of an ideal liquid culture medium (ie ascites) in their peritoneal space.

5 **Hypoglycaemia.** Normally the liver acts as a store for glycogen, from which glucose can readily be liberated if the need arises. In chronic liver failure, little glycogen is stored in the damaged organ and therefore the patient is susceptible to significant hypoglycaemia if their blood sugar level falls.

6 **Hepatorenal syndrome.** This is a functional renal failure that can occur in patients with advanced liver disease. Its exact cause is unknown, but it may be related to failure of the liver to break down the toxins that cause reno-vascular shutdown. The patient develops the features of acute pre-renal renal failure, with oliguria and rapidly rising creatinine levels. This condition has an extremely poor prognosis.

Gastrointestinal disorders

CASE
42

💊 Treatment

In cases of chronic liver disease every effort must be made to prevent any further damage to the liver. Patients must abstain from alcohol, hepatotoxic drugs must be stopped, and aggressive treatment of any underlying disease process must be started. Every effort should be made to reduce the development of hepatic encephalopathy and hypoglycaemia by adopting a low-protein, high-carbohydrate dietary regime. Infections should be promptly treated with appropriate antibiotics. Endoscopy should be performed to identify the presence of oesophageal varices, and these must be treated by sclerotherapy or oesophageal banding to reduce the risk of bleeding. Assessment of the patient's coagulation status should be carried out by measuring the prothrombin time, and if the latter is prolonged, vitamin K supplementation should be given to encourage the production of clotting factors.

If despite every effort there is evidence of progressive liver failure, the only hope of cure is by liver transplantation. This is performed at specialist centres, and the patient must be referred for assessment at a stage when they are in a reasonable state of health, which is necessary if they are to successfully undergo this very major procedure.

Gastrointestinal disorders

CASE
42

CASE 43

Hepatitis

This condition will most often be encountered at a data interpretation station, where the student is asked to interpret abnormal liver function test results and then answer questions about the diagnosis, investigation and treatment of hepatitis.

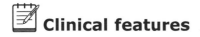 Definition

Hepatitis is inflammation of the liver, which causes damage to and loss of function of the hepatocytes.

Hepatitis may be acute or chronic, and the causes are as follows:

1 Acute hepatitis:
   - viral hepatitis
   - alcohol-induced
   - bacterial infection
   - haemochromatosis.

2 Chronic hepatitis:
   - autoimmune disease
   - chronic viral infection
   - Wilson's disease
   - drug-induced.

Clinical features

Viral hepatitis

The common viral infections of the liver are hepatitis A, B and C, cytomegalovirus and some adenoviruses. Irrespective of the type of virus that causes the infection, the clinical features are broadly similar. There is a prodromal period of flu-like symptoms with fever, malaise, anorexia and nausea, and there may be associated muscle aches and pains. The patient then develops jaundice accompanied by

CASE
43

darkening of the urine, and later the stools may become pale. Symptoms may persist for a variable period, but usually resolve within two to four weeks. Treatment is symptomatic; bed rest and avoidance of fatty foods are usually advocated.

The type of virus that is causing the infection can be determined by serological testing, which identifies specific antiviral antibody responses during the course of the illness. An initial rise in viral-specific IgM followed by a rise in viral-specific IgG is diagnostic. The different hepatitis viruses have differing modes of transmission and incubation periods (see Table 10).

Table 10 Incubation period, mode of transmission and prognosis of infection with hepatitis A, B and C viruses

	A virus (50%)	B virus (30%)	C virus (20%)
Incubation period	3–6 weeks	1–4 months	2–8 weeks
Mode of transmission	Faecal/oral	By inoculation or sexual contact	By transfusion By transfusion Blood products
Prognosis	Good	20% chronic infection	> 80% chronic carriers who develop cirrhosis

In all cases, during the acute phase of the illness the liver function tests show evidence of hepatocellular damage with release of transaminase enzymes. The serum levels of aspartate aminotransferase (AST) and alanine aminotranferase (ALT) rise. Because the hepatocytes are unable to conjugate bilirubin, the serum level of unconjugated bilirubin also rises. Only if the inflammation in the liver is sufficient to cause some degree of obstruction of the bile canaliculi does the alkaline phosphatase level rise.

Due to the liver cell dysfunction, the production of vitamin K-dependent clotting factors decreases and the prothrombin time will increase. This is a useful marker of severity of disease, and serial measurements can be used to monitor progression or recovery.

Gastrointestinal disorders

CASE
43

Chronic hepatitis

This can occur as a result of a number of autoimmune disorders, chronic viral infection (especially hepatitis B or C), in association with inflammatory bowel disease (especially ulcerative colitis), as a result of infection spreading up the biliary system from the bowel (ascending cholangitis), or may be due to disorders of copper or iron metabolism (eg Wilson's disease, haemochromatosis).

Patients may initially have clinical features associated with the primary underlying disorder, but then develop jaundice and clinical features of chronic liver failure or cirrhosis. The clinical signs of chronic liver disease are shown in Table 9 on page 113.

The main aim of therapy is to treat the underlying disease process to prevent further liver cell inflammation or damage. Anti-inflammatory drugs, particularly steroids and immunosuppressive drugs, are used to treat autoimmune disorders. If liver cell damage and cirrhosis develop to the extent that the patient is at risk of developing hepatic encephalopathy, liver transplantation must be considered as the only means of effecting a cure.

Gastrointestinal disorders

CASE
43

Haematology

CASE 44

The tired patient

Tiredness and lack of energy are two of the commonest complaints that patients describe when they consult their general practitioner. These problems can be associated with a wide variety of organic, psychosomatic and psychiatric disorders.

A history-taking station with a simulated patient complaining of tiredness is an excellent challenge for students.

Definition

It is important to determine exactly what the patient means when they complain of tiredness, as there are three major conditions which can be considered as tiredness:

1 sleepiness or lassitude – this is the desire to sleep, and it is often associated with failure to derive benefit from sleep

2 lack of energy or listlessness – this is the feeling that one has insufficient energy to complete the normal tasks of daily living

3 weakness – this is a reduction in muscle power. It may be localised to one or several muscle groups, or it may be generalised.

Often a combination of these conditions occurs together in any given patient.

? Causes of tiredness

These can be classified as follows:

1 Haematological causes:
- anaemia due to iron deficiency, vitamin B_{12} deficiency, haemoglobinopathies, haemoloytic disease or hereditary cell defects
- leukaemia/lymphoma.

2 Renal causes:
- renal failure with or without electrolyte disorders.

Haematology

CASE 44

3 Endocrine/metabolic causes:

- hypothyroidism
- acromegaly
- adrenal insufficiency
- hypopituitarism
- haemochromatosis.

4 Neuromuscular causes:

- myasthenia gravis
- myotonia
- motor neurone disease
- Parkinson's disease
- polymyositis.

5 Cardiovascular causes:

- left ventricular failure
- ischaemic heart disease
- aortic valve disease
- mitral valve disease
- cardiomyopathy.

6. Other causes:

- post-viral fatigue syndrome
- chronic fatigue syndrome.

Psychosomatic causes

As a result of emotional stress or conflict, patients frequently complain of a variety of symptoms, including tiredness and/or weakness, for which no cause can be found.

Psychiatric causes

Depression is usually associated with feelings of tiredness and lethargy.

CASE
44

Clinical features

It is important to determine from the history and examination which of the three conditions – lassitude, lack of energy and/or muscle weakness – the patient is experiencing. If objective evidence of muscle weakness is not detected, neurological causes can usually be ruled out. A series of simple laboratory investigations can then be used to identify the presence or absence of an underlying organic disorder.

Investigations

Full blood picture

Look for evidence of anaemia. The features of the red cells, including their size and shape, and the mean corpuscular haemoglobin concentration may give a clue to the aetiology of anaemia, if present. The total and differential white cell count may indicate underlying haematological malignancy or bone marrow infiltration.

Biochemical analysis

Electrolyte disorders, such as hyponatraemia, hypokalaemia, hypocalcaemia and renal failure can all cause tiredness and lethargy. The levels of urea and creatinine will indicate the presence of significant underlying renal impairment.

Endocrine tests

Abnormal thyroid function tests – that is, low free thyroxine (T4) and elevated thyroid-stimulating hormone (TSH) levels – indicate primary hypothyroidism. A low T4 and low TSH might indicate hypopituitarism and warrant dynamic pituitary function tests.

Postural hypotension and hyponatraemia

In a tired patient, these findings are suggestive of adrenal insufficiency. If the random cortisol level is low, a Synacthen[R] (ACTH) stimulation test should be performed. If hypoadrenalism is secondary to hypopituitarism, the ACTH level will be low.

Growth hormone assay

This should be performed if the clinical features are suggestive of acromegaly.

Haematology

CASE
44

Serum and urinary immunoglobulins

With electrophoresis these may indicate the presence of a paraprotein or immunoparesis, which may be associated with myeloma or lymphoma.

Serum iron levels

Total iron-binding capacity and ferritin levels will reveal any iron-deficiency state or haemochromatosis.

Serum vitamin B_{12} and folate levels

These will usually confirm the cause of a macrocytic hyperchromic anaemia, although a bone marrow aspirate showing megaloblastic change is sometimes needed for confirmation.

Cardiovascular causes can usually be diagnosed from the history and clinical findings, with valvular defects and left ventricular insufficiency confirmed by echocardiography.

Haematology

CASE 44

CASE 45

The anaemic patient

Anaemia is a common medical condition, and may be either a primary disorder or secondary to some other underlying disease state.

Definition and classification

Anaemia is defined as a reduction in haemoglobin concentration below the normal range for an age/sex-matched population.

Anaemia can be classified according to the underlying aetiological cause as follows:

1 reduced blood cell formation due to a deficiency of essential haematinic factors

2 bone marrow suppression

3 excessive blood loss or red cell destruction.

Deficiency of essential factors

Any deficiency of essential haematinics, such as iron, vitamin B_{12}, folate, protein or vitamin C, will result in anaemia. The deficiency may be the result of a reduced intake in the diet, reduced absorption due to an underlying malabsorption syndrome, increased losses of these essential haematinic substances, or reduced utilisation of haematinics by the bone marrow.

Iron deficiency is the commonest cause of anaemia. It may be due to reduced dietary intake, malabsorption of dietary iron or chronic blood loss. The clinical features that suggest iron deficiency as a cause of anaemia include glossitis, angular stomatitis, brittle nails and koilonychia. The patient may give a history suggestive of excessive or chronic blood loss. Iron deficiency anaemia is particularly common in women with menorrhagia.

The blood picture will reveal a hypochromic microcytic anaemia. The total serum iron concentration will be reduced, iron-binding capacity will be increased and the ferritin level will be markedly lowered.

Haematology

CASE 45

Vitamin B_{12} deficiency anaemia causes a hyperchromic macrocytic anaemia, and the bone marrow is megaloblastic. It is associated with vitamin B_{12} deficiency as a result of reduced dietary intake, malabsorption, blind loop syndrome or pernicious anaemia. Other clinical features that may be present are those associated with peripheral neuropathy or altered function of the posterior columns of the spinal chord, such as reduced vibration sensation in the lower limbs and altered proprioception.

Reduced red cell formation

Any condition that suppresses bone marrow activity can result in anaemia. This will be reflected not only in a reduced red cell count and haemoglobin level, but also in a reduction in the white cell and platelet counts (pancytopenia). It may occur as a result of chronic infection, major organ failure (eg renal failure), liver disease, malignant disease or some chronic inflammatory conditions (eg rheumatoid arthritis). However, the commonest cause is bone marrow suppression secondary to the use of cytotoxic drugs.

Excessive blood loss or red cell destruction

Anaemia occurs as a result of either overt blood loss or occult blood loss in the urine or faeces. It also occurs in conditions where there is excessive red cell destruction, such as congenital red cell abnormalities (eg spherocytosis) or hereditary haemoglobinopathies, and it can occur as an autoimmune disorder (eg autoimmune haemolytic anaemia) or secondary to any condition that causes splenomegaly.

Investigations

Investigation of anaemia involves obtaining a full blood picture. The morphology of the red cells may give a clue to the underlying cause. Measurement of essential haematimic factors such as iron, vitamin B_{12} and folate, and biochemical analyses to rule out underlying major organ disease are first-line investigations. However, bone-marrow aspiration and trephine biopsy may be necessary to establish a diagnosis.

Treatment

Therapy is aimed at treating the underlying cause and rectifying any deficiency state which may be present.

CASE
45

CASE 46

The patient who bruises or bleeds easily

The presence of spontaneous bleeding or easy bruising is often a sign of serious underlying pathology, and it is vital that students are familiar with the underlying causes and know how to investigate patients with these symptoms.

? Causes

Any deficiency or dysfunction of platelets or of the coagulation cascade will affect the homeostatic mechanism that prevents bruising or bleeding.

Platelet disorders

The platelets are responsible for preventing loss of blood from normal blood vessels. Any deficiency in number of platelets (thrombocytopenia) or abnormality of platelet function (eg a defect in platelet aggregation) will result in features of spontaneous bleeds in the skin, namely petechiae (1–2 mm), purpura (2–20 mm) or ecchymoses (> 20 mm). Patients may develop spontaneous bruising (ie development of a bruise with no history of trauma), bleeding from the gums, nosebleeds, haematemesis or haemoptysis. Platelet numbers are normally 150–400 x 10^9/l, and spontaneous bleeding will only develop when the platelet count falls below 10 x 10^9/l. Platelet deficiency may occur as a result of any of the following:

1 Bone marrow suppression:

- cytotoxic or chemotherapeutic drugs
- excess alcohol consumption
- radiation exposure
- side effects of therapeutic drugs.

2 Bone marrow infiltration:

- leukaemia/lymphoma
- multiple myeloma
- secondary malignancy.

Haematology

CASE
46

3 Autoimmune disease:
- systemic lupus erythematosus – antiplatelet antibodies
- hypersplenism.

4 Disseminated intravascular coagulation:
- infection
- malignancy.

Abnormal platelet function

In some patients the number of platelets is normal or may even be increased, but there is defective platelet aggregation or activation of the coagulation cascade. This may occur especially in myelodysplasia or myelofibrosis. Chronic renal failure is associated with platelet dysfunction.

The Hess test

This test is performed using a sphygmomanometer. The cuff is inflated to just above systolic pressure and left for two minutes. If there is a defect in platelet function or thrombocytopenia, small petechial haemorrhages appear in the skin of the arm and hand below the level of the cuff. Certain drugs, especially aspirin or aspirin-containing drug compounds, inhibit platelet aggregation and can cause platelet dysfunction.

Disorders of clotting factors

These include the following:

1 Hereditary disorders:
- haemophilia
- von Willebrand's disease
- Christmas disease.
2 Drugs – patients on anticoagulants.
3 Liver disease – chronic liver failure or acute liver damage (eg paracetamol overdose) results in a deficiency of factors II, VII, IX, XI and protein C and protein S (vitamin K-dependent clotting factors).
4 Malabsorption – as vitamin K is a fat-soluble vitamin, any cause of fat malabsorption will result in vitamin K deficiency and this can lead to a deficiency of vitamin K-dependent clotting factors.

Haematology (sidebar)

CASE
46

Investigations

1 Full blood picture, differential white cell count and platelet count, to rule out thrombocytopenia and leukaemia.

2 If the platelet count is normal or increased, platelet function tests should be requested.

3 Liver function tests, including prothrombin time.

4 Serum immunoglobulins and urine for Bence Jones proteins, to rule out multiple myeloma and lymphoma.

5 Clotting factor assay.

6 Screening tests for malabsorption.

7 Bone marrow aspirate and trephine biopsy may be necessary to determine the nature of the bone marrow defect.

Haematology

CASE
46

CASE 47

Lymphoma

Lymphomas may be encountered at clinical stations where there are patients with obvious lymph node enlargement. Alternatively, they may be seen in data interpretation stations where the student is presented with the results of serum immunoglobulin tests, or in radiology stations with a chest X-ray showing mediastinal lymphadenopathy.

Definition and classification

Lymphoma is a malignant condition that affects the lymphoid series of cells and causes enlargement of lymphatic tissue, particularly in the lymph nodes and/or the spleen.

Lymphomas can be classified as Hodgkin's lymphoma or non-Hodgkin's lymphoma.

Non-Hodgkin's lymphomas can in turn be subdivided into two types:

1 diffuse – which can be subdivided into lymphocytic, histiocytic and mixed types.
2 nodular – which can be subdivided into lymphocytic, histiocytic, mixed, Burkitt's lymphoma and undifferentiated (stem cell) types.

This classification system is based on the histological appearance of the lymph nodes at the time of biopsy.

Clinical features

The commonest form of presentation is painless enlargement of one or more lymph nodes with no other symptoms. However, in some patients there is fever with night sweats, weight loss, itching or pain after drinking alcohol. In 20% of patients splenomegaly is present, and it is more common in the lymphocytic varieties of non-Hodgkin's lymphoma. Mediastinal lymph nodes occur in 20% of patients. Intrathoracic disease may present with features of superior vena caval obstruction or pleural effusion.

CASE
47

Investigations

The most useful investigations are lymph node biopsy and histology which confirms the diagnosis. Other investigations that can be helpful are chest X-ray (which may show paratracheal or mediastinal lymphadenopathy) and serum immunoglobulins (which can show either a rise in paraprotein levels if the malignant transformation is occurring in B lymphocytes, causing the production of a monoclonal antibody, or immunoparesis, which results from the malignant clone of cells impairing normal B cell proliferation and thus causing a secondary hypogammaglobulinaemia).

Treatment

Treatment of the condition depends on the stage of the disease, and this requires radiological imaging (usually CT or MRI scans) to determine the extent of the condition.

- Stage 1 – a single lymph node region or a single extralymphatic site is affected
- Stage 2 – two or more lymph node regions are affected on the same side of the diaphragm
- Stage 3 – two or more lymph node regions are affected on both sides of the diaphragm
- Stage 4 – there is diffuse involvement of lymph nodes and extralymphatic sites.

Each stage can be subdivided into A or B, where A is lymph node enlargement only and B is lymph node enlargement together with associated symptoms of sweating, itching or alcohol-induced pain.

Treatment for stages 1 and 2 is local radiotherapy to the involved node sites, and this usually results in a good response. For stages 3 and 4 chemotherapy is required, although occasionally radiotherapy is also used to reduce the size of the nodes, particularly if they are causing any obstructive symptoms.

The prognosis very much depends on the stage and histological type of the tumour. A better prognosis is associated with Hodgkin's lymphoma and well-differentiated lymphocytic tumours.

Haematology

CASE
47

CASE 48

Leukaemia

In an OSCE examination the topic of leukaemia may arise either during the clinical examination of a patient with an enlarged spleen or lymphadenopathy, or at a data interpretation station where the student is given a full blood picture result with a differential white cell count from a patient with a form of leukaemia.

Definition and types

Leukaemia is the malignant transformation and proliferation of cells of either the myeloid or lymphoid cell lines in the bone marrow.

There are four types of leukaemia:

1 acute lymphatic leukaemia
2 chronic lymphatic leukaemia
3 acute myeloid leukaemia
4 chronic myeloid leukaemia.

Acute lymphatic leukaemia affects children, chronic lymphatic leukaemia affects the elderly, and both acute and chronic myeloid leukaemias affect young adults.

Acute lymphatic leukaemia

This is the common form of leukaemia seen in young children. It usually presents with symptoms of anaemia with tiredness and lack of energy, and on clinical examination the child may be found to have lymphadenopathy.

Investigations show the presence of large numbers of immature lymphocytes in the circulation due to the proliferation of lymphoblasts in the bone marrow. Patients usually respond well to chemotherapy, and the prognosis is good.

Haematology

CASE 48

Chronic lymphatic leukaemia

This is a condition mainly of old age. Patients may present with symptoms of anaemia, bleeding disorder or the development of lymphadenopathy. Examination usually reveals the presence of firm lymph nodes scattered in various lymph node regions of the body. There may or may not be slight splenomegaly or liver enlargement.

On investigation, the white cell count is found to be elevated due to the presence of large numbers of mature lymphocytes. In most cases (97%) the malignant transformation occurs in B lymphocytes and the patient may have a detectable paraprotein circulating in the blood. This condition is slowly progressive and can usually be kept well controlled with chemotherapy.

Acute and chronic myeloid leukaemia

Both of these conditions involve a malignant transformation of the myeloid series of cells in the bone marrow, and both are extremely serious. They usually affect young adults, who present with symptoms of anaemia or a bleeding disorder, or are detected at the time of presentation with infection. On examination these patients are often found to have marked splenomegaly. The bone marrow is replaced with a malignant transformation of myeloid cells, which in chronic myeloid leukaemia are recognised as precursors of the granulocytes of blood. Chronic myeloid leukaemia can change into an acute myeloid disorder in which the cells become large and have the appearance of myeloblasts and metamyelocytes. This condition is not very responsive to chemotherapy, and the mainstay of treatment is an aggressive chemotherapeutic regime. The only treatment that offers hope of long-term survival is bone marrow transplantation.

Haematology

CASE
48

CASE 49

Multiple myeloma

This condition is most likely to be encountered in a data interpretation station. The abnormalities are usually related to calcium metabolism, serum immunoglobulins or urinary proteins.

Definition

Multiple myeloma is a malignant proliferation of plasma cells, usually occurring within the bone marrow and manifested by widespread destruction of the bone, associated with anaemia, hypercalcaemia, impaired renal function and the production of monoclonal antibody or immunoglobulin light chains.

? Causes

This condition affects men and women equally and can occur in all age groups, although the peak incidence is in those aged 50–60 years.

Clinical features

Initially the disease may be asymptomatic for many months or years, but then the patient can develop a variety of symptoms, most commonly due to anaemia resulting from replacement of bone marrow with the plasma cell proliferation. They may also develop pains in the bones, pathological fractures or features of hypercalcaemia.

On clinical examination the patient may have bony tenderness, particularly over the sternum, there may be features of anaemia, and investigations reveal a raised erythrocyte sedimentation rate (often in excess of 100 mm in the first hour). Serum immunoglobulins show a monoclonal band of immunoglobulin which is often described as an M band ('M' for monoclonal), although the immunoglobulin class that is involved is most commonly IgG, but may be IgA or IgM. The patient may excrete large quantities of immunoglobulin light chains in the urine (these are known as Bence Jones proteins). A bone profile often shows features of a secondary malignancy with increased serum calcium levels and increased alkaline phosphatase activity. X-rays may show either generalised osteoporosis or lytic lesions, which appear as 'punched out' areas of radiolucency that are especially obvious in the bones of the skull and the pelvis.

CASE 49

Haematology

Diagnosis is made on the basis of three out of four diagnostic criteria:

1 a serum paraprotein concentration of > 4 g/litre
2 the presence of Bence Jones proteins in the urine
3 lytic lesions on bone X-ray
4 an increased number of plasma cells in the bone marrow aspirate (> 4% of the nucleated cells).

Treatment

Patients are treated with busulfan, which is an alkylating agent that can be used over a period of many months or years to keep the condition under control. Disease activity is monitored by measuring the erythrocyte sedimentation rate and the level of paraprotein in the blood.

Death may occur as a result of renal failure due to the renal tubules becoming blocked by the high levels of protein, or as a consequence of secondary amyloidosis. It is important that patients maintain a high fluid intake in order to prevent the development of renal failure, and hypercalcaemia must be treated appropriately.

With adequate hydration, the use of cytotoxic drugs such as alkylating agents or cyclophosphamide and control of hypercalcaemia, 80% of patients achieve remission for a number of years.

Haematology

CASE
49

Nervous system

CASE 50

The patient with headache

Headache is an extremely common complaint which affects nearly everyone at least occasionally, and is estimated to be a problem at some time in the lives of 40% of people in the UK. It is therefore a frequent cause of consultation and provides a useful history-taking session to assess the student's ability to take a history and differentiate between the more common and more serious causes of the condition.

? Causes

The list of causes of headache is extensive, and includes benign conditions such as tension headache, migraine, alcohol withdrawal states and eye strain. However, there are a number of serious underlying conditions which must be considered in any patient who presents with headache. These include meningitis, subarachnoid haemorrhage, raised intracranial pressure due to space-occupying lesions, brain abscess, cerebrovascular events, giant-cell arteritis (temporal arteritis) and hypertension.

When taking a history It is useful to ask the following questions:

1 **Exact site of pain.** Is it localised, generalised, unilateral or bilateral?

2 **Duration.** Has the headache been present for a long period of time or Is it an acute headache? Is it constant or periodic? How long does each episode of pain last?

3 **Character of pain.** The character of the pain often reflects the underlying cause. For example, vascular headaches are more likely to be throbbing in nature, while space-occupying lesions cause constant pain or pressure that is felt inside the head.

4 **Severity of pain.** This should be quantified on a scale of 0–10, where 0 is no pain and 10 is the most severe pain that the patient has ever experienced. However, severity of pain may not correlate with the seriousness of the underlying cause, as patients with raised intracranial pressure or large tumours may not experience severe pain.

5 **Triggering factors.** The patient should be asked about factors that bring on the pain or aggravate It, such as straining, bending forward, coughing or sneezing, or exposure to light.

Nervous system

CASE 50

6 **Associated symptoms.** The patient should be asked about associated symptoms, such as any change in visual acuity, the presence or absence of fortification spectra (zigzag lines), nausea, vomiting or photophobia.

7 **State of health between attacks.** It is important to ascertain whether or not the patient is completely well or has any symptoms between headaches, and also to determine what concerns or anxieties they may have about the cause of their symptoms.

Conditions that cause acute headache and which must be considered include the following:

- subarachnoid haemorrhage
- cerebrovascular accident
- meningitis
- giant-cell arteritis (temporal arteritis)
- idiopathic intracranial hypertension
- hypertensive encephalopathy
- intracranial lesions presenting as an acute event, such as a bleed into a tumour.

Clinical features

Clinical signs that should be assessed in all patients with headache include body temperature, pulse and blood pressure, mental state and evidence of disorientation, confusion, and altered higher cerebral function, such as short-term memory or concentration. The patient's relatives should be asked about any change in personality or behaviour. All patients should have a full neurological examination, focusing in particular on cranial nerve examination and assessment of the fundi, looking for papilloedema (raised intracranial pressure) or evidence of hypertensive retinopathy. Clinical features associated with the underlying cause may also be present.

Treatment

This will depend on the underlying condition that needs to be treated, together with analgesia.

CASE
50

CASE 51

Falls, fits, faints and funny turns

There are many reasons why patients collapse, and this is a very good station for assessing the student's history-taking skills and reasoning ability in trying to identify the underlying cause of a relatively common clinical problem.

Definition

Collapse is an involuntary event which results in the patient falling to the ground due to an inability to maintain an upright posture.

? Causes

These can be thought of as the four F's, namely falls, fits, faints and funny turns!

Falls

These are characterised by the fact that the collapse occurs before consciousness is lost, and by an absence of preceding symptoms. Usually there is no loss of consciousness unless there is a significant head injury subsequent to the fall. Falls can occur due to simple accidents (eg tripping over a mat, falling down stairs). However, some underlying disorders may predispose to falls (eg hemiparesis, multiple sclerosis, hemianopia, parkinsonism), and all of these disorders can affect mobility or increase the risk of accidental falls.

Drop attacks

These are characterised by sudden loss of power in the lower limbs, and are caused by a reduction in the blood supply in the spinal arteries, which supply the spinal cord. There are usually no preceding symptoms, and the patient suddenly falls to the ground due to an abrupt loss of power in the legs. There is no loss of consciousness, and the patient has total recall of the event.

Nervous system

CASE 51

Fits

Epileptic seizures (fits) occur as a result of spontaneous electrical activity in the brain disrupting normal function. In most cases consciousness is lost and a variety of manifestations can occur. It is extremely important to obtain a reliable eyewitness account of the events, as this is essential for diagnosis.

Types of fit

- Tonic-clonic seizures – these may be preceded by an aura, followed by sudden loss of consciousness with collapse. The tonic phase of muscle contraction is followed by the tonic-clonic phase, with rhythmic jerking of the limbs, biting of the tongue, loss of continence and post-ictal confusion.

- Absence seizures – there is loss of consciousness for brief periods (5–10 seconds), but the eyes remain open and staring, and there is no collapse.

- Partial seizures – there is abnormal electrical activity that causes involuntary jerking of a limb or part of a limb, and which can progress to tonic-clonic seizures. In simple partial seizures the patient remains conscious throughout, while in complex partial seizures consciousness is lost and an episode of collapse will occur.

Faints

Vasovagal episodes

These are relatively common, especially in adolescent females. They only occur when the patient is standing up, and they may be triggered by emotion or a prolonged period of standing. The patient describes a sinking sensation, they feel cold and clammy, and then they fall to the floor. There is usually no involuntary movement, tongue biting or loss of continence. A bradycardia is present during the event. Consciousness is quickly regained as the cerebral blood flow is restored by lying flat.

Postural hypotension

This is defined as dizziness, faintness or collapse due to a drop in systolic blood pressure resulting from standing up after being in a sitting or lying position. It may be accompanied by a tachycardia. Postural hypotension is diagnosed by demonstrating a drop in systolic pressure of more than 10 mmHg between supine and standing blood pressure recordings.

Nervous system

CASE
51

There are various causes, including cardiac arrhythmias, left ventricular failure, hypovolaemia, autonomic neuropathy and the side effects of certain drugs (eg antihypertensive drugs).

Funny turns

A patient may fall to the ground for a variety of reasons, and usually there are one or more preceding symptoms which give a clue to the cause. The term 'funny turn' derives from the fact that the patient usually states that they feel funny (ie strange or unusual) before they collapse. Funny turns may or may not be associated with loss of consciousness. The common preceding symptoms or events include the following:

- palpitations – indicating that a cardiac rhythm disturbance is the possible underlying cause
- vertigo/tinnitus – indicating an ENT problem, such as labyrinthitis or Ménière's disease
- head movement – suggesting vertebrobasilar insufficiency
- use of an upper limb – subclavian steal syndrome
- reflex syncope – micturition, cough, emotional state
- vertigo – Ménière's disease, benign positional, vestibular neuronitis, labyrinthitis
- psychogenic symptoms – hyperventilation, panic attack, pseudoseizures
- metabolic and endocrine causes – hyper- or hypoglycaemia, phaeochromocytoma, carcinoid syndrome.

Nervous system

CASE
51

CASE 52

Transient ischaemic attack

A large number of conditions can lead to transient ischaemic attack, and this is frequently encountered at a history-taking station that is used to test the student's ability to discriminate between the more common causes of the attack.

📖 Definition

Transient ischaemic attack is a transient neurological abnormality or deficit which resolves completely within 24 hours.

❓ Causes

It may be caused by any condition that results in a transient drop in blood pressure or blockage of a branch of the cerebral circulation so that a reversible area of cerebral ischaemia occurs sufficient to cause a neurological event. There is complete recovery on reperfusion of the affected area.

The commonest causes are as follows:

- embolism (80%) – platelet emboli from atheromatous plaques in the carotid or vertebral arterial circulation.
- embolism from the heart (20%) – left atrial thrombus, atrial myxoma (rare), vegetation on mitral or aortic valves (bacterial endocarditis).

📝 Clinical features

The patient is usually completely fit and well and then suddenly develops a neurological deficit, such as loss of power or sensation in one limb or part of a limb, a speech disorder (eg dysphasia or dysarthria), a visual field defect or an isolated cranial nerve paralysis. The neurological deficit is usually maximal shortly after the onset and then recovers rapidly, being fully resolved within 24 hours. The features of the focal neurological abnormality can help to identify the area of cerebral artery where the deficiency or occlusion has occurred (see Table 11).

CASE
52

Table 11 Relationship between the symptoms of transient ischaemic attack and arterial distribution

Symptom	Arterial distribution
Speech disorder	Carotid, dominant hemisphere
Visual loss of one eye	Carotid, same side
Weakness of face, arm or leg	Carotid, opposite side
Dysarthria or slurring	Carotid or vertebrobasilar
Sensory loss in face, arm or leg	Carotid, opposite side
Hemianopia	Vertebrobasilar
Bilateral blindness	Vertebrobasilar
Double vision	Vertebrobasilar

If the cause is an arrhythmia, the patient may have preceding symptoms of palpitations or chest pain.

Patients often have a history of previous attacks, and again the features of these may give some clue to the cause and/or site of origin of the disorder. For example, if the episodes are identical or very similar, always involving a speech defect, the embolus must be originating from a branch of the carotid artery supplying Broca's area of the dominant hemisphere. If each neurological event is different but clearly always represents a disorder occurring in the same cerebral hemisphere, such as left-sided facial weakness followed some months later by sensory loss in the left leg and foot, followed some weeks later by loss of vision in the right eye, then embolism from a plaque in the right internal carotid artery would seem most likely. If events affect both cerebral hemispheres and areas supplied by the carotid and vertebrobasilar arteries, then embolism arising from within the heart or aorta is more likely, with emboli moving at random into various branches of the arterial tree.

Investigations

Doppler studies of the carotid and vertebrobasilar arteries will show whether or not there is narrowing or significant plaque formation which could be a source for platelet emboli to aggregate and then break off.

Echocardiography (either transthoracic or transoesphageal) can be used to identify the presence of blood clot, myxoma in the left atrium or the presence of vegetations on the mitral or aortic valves. If endocarditis is suspected, blood cultures should be

Nervous system

CASE
52

performed, and of course inflammatory markers such as the white cell count, erythrocyte sedimentation rate and C-reactive protein will be raised.

Cardiac arrhythmias that could cause transient hypotension may be revealed by 24-hour ECG monitoring.

Treatment

Since, by definition, there is complete recovery from these neurological events, the main aims of treatment are to prevent further attacks and to endeavour to prevent a more serious cerebrovascular accident from taking place. Patients should be given low-dose aspirin, 75 mg daily, to reduce platelet adhesion and prevent the formation of platelet aggregates.

This treatment must not be given to patients with a history of aspirin hypersensitivity or if contraindicated (eg in patients with a past history of aspirin-induced peptic ulceration or gastritis). Alternative antiplatelet drugs such as dipyridamole or clopidogrel are available for use in such patients.

If carotid Doppler studies indicate critical narrowing due to artheroma, surgical endarterectomy may be needed. If thrombus is detected in the left atrium, anticoagulation with warfarin is required, provided that there is no contraindication.

Patients with bacterial endocarditis should be treated appropriately with antibiotic therapy, which usually results in resolution of the vegetations. Occasionally it is necessary to perform cardiac valve replacement surgery.

If the transient ischaemic attacks are due to episodes of arrhythmia, anti-arrhythmic drugs or cardiac pacemaker therapy is indicated to correct the rhythm disturbance.

Nervous system

CASE
52

CASE 53

Cerebrovascular accidents and hemiparesis

Students are expected to be able to examine patients with power and/or sensory loss. These common conditions are used to assess clinical examination skills and are frequently encountered at an examination station.

Definition

Cerebrovascular accidents may occur for a number of reasons, but the end result is permanent damage to an area of the central nervous system, causing neurological deficit. This may be loss of power, loss of sensation, cranial nerve damage, loss of speech, or a combination of any of these.

? Causes

Permanent neurological damage occurs as a result of interruption of the blood supply to any part of the brain, which can be due to thrombosis, embolism or haemorrhage. It can also occur if there is abnormal tissue present, such as primary or secondary tumour, inflammatory tissue or an abscess.

The majority of cerebrovascular accidents occur as a result of emboli from atheromatous plaques or thrombus formation in arteriosclerotic branches of the cerebral arterial circulation. Risk factors for both ischaemic and haemorrhagic cerebrovascular accidents include the following:

- hypertension
- cigarette smoking
- diabetes mellitus
- positive family history
- hyperlipidaemia.

Although cerebrovascular accidents can occur at any age, they usually affect older individuals, who often have clinical features associated with the risk factors listed above.

Nervous system

CASE 53

Causes of cerebrovascular accidents can be summarised as follows:

1 Ischaemic causes (80%):

- embolism (80%) – fibrin and platelet embolus, is usually arising on an atheromatous plaque of the internal carotid or vertebrobasilar artery
- thrombosis (20%) – occlusion of a branch of the cerebral arterial system.

2 Haemorrhagic cause (15%):

- arterial rupture (10%) or rupture of a berry aneurysm or arteriovenous malformation (5%).

3 Other causes (5%):

- primary or secondary tumour with or without haemorrhage
- brain abscess
- granulomatous disease
- infection
- giant-cell arteritis
- polyarteritis nodosa.

If a cerebrovascular accident occurs in a young person, one should suspect either the rupture of a berry aneurysm or some of the rarer underlying causes, such as systemic lupus erythematosus, polyarteritis or an infective process.

The majority of patients have sudden onset of a neurological deficit, which may be focal (eg affecting one limb) or can be more extensive (eg complete paralysis of the arm and leg on one side of the body). The type of neurological deficit is determined by which region of the central nervous system has its blood supply interrupted.

For ischaemic and haemorrhagic strokes, the onset is abrupt and maximal features occur at an early stage, usually within hours.

Strokes associated with tumours are less abrupt in onset, and often the neurological features progressively worsen over a period of days or weeks as the tumour expands, or as a result of oedematous swelling of the surrounding brain tissue. The commonest form of ischaemic cerebrovascular accident affects the middle cerebral arterial system and causes paralysis of the arm and leg on the opposite side

Nervous system

CASE
53

(hemiplegia), or reduced power of those limbs (hemiparesis). Power is absent or reduced, and initially muscle tone is reduced (hypotonia), but within 24 to 48 hours the tone increases and hypertonia develops. Reflexes become brisk and abnormal reflexes may be elicited (eg finger jerk and Hoffman's jerk in the hand and extensor plantar response in the foot) on the affected side. Abnormalities of speech (aphasia or dysphasia) will occur if the event occurs in the dominant hemisphere and involves Broca's area or the association areas of the speech centre.

Sensory loss and/or facial nerve weakness (upper motor neurone lesion) will be present if the sensory areas or region of cerebral cortex which represents the face are involved.

Investigations

CT or MRI scans are extremely important for three reasons:

1 to confirm the diagnosis – they show the area of necrosis of the central nervous system

2 to differentiate between ischaemic and haemorrhagic stroke – if the patient has an ischaemic stroke (embolism or thrombus), thrombolytic, antiplatelet or anticoagulant drugs might be considered. However, if the event was due to haemorrhage it would be extremely dangerous to consider using thrombolytic therapy or anticoagulation

3 to look for other underlying pathology, such as primary or secondary tumours, berry aneurysms, areas of infection or abscess formation.

Other investigations can be performed to rule out other underlying diseases such as systemic lupus erythematosus or vasculitis.

Treatment

Early treatment

Supportive treatment is used in the early stages, with intravenous fluids, oxygen and expert nursing care.

Specific therapy depends on the underlying cause:

- embolism – antiplatelet therapy
- thrombosis – thrombolytic therapy/anticoagulation
- haemorrhage – may require surgical drainage.

Nervous system

CASE 53

Subsequent treatment

Once the event has been adequately managed, the main aim is to maximise the recovery of power and function. Recovery can take many months, and depends on expert nursing care, physiotherapy and occupational therapy, with a great deal of effort and co-operation from the patient and their family. Patients can continue to recover for up to two years after the acute event. However, they will have an increased risk of another cerebrovascular accident within the first year (10%), and the annual risk thereafter is 5%. It is vitally important that any contributing risk factors are identified and, where possible, reduced.

Nervous system

CASE 54

The confused patient

Confusion is a common medical problem that is often seen in elderly patients. It is important that the student is aware of the causes of confusion and how to recognise and manage an acute confusional state.

Definition

A person is said to be confused if they are not fully orientated in time, place and person and not functioning to their full intellectual capacity, or have impaired cognitive function.

? Causes

There are two main types of confusional state:

1 chronic confusional state – most commonly due to Alzheimer's disease (senile dementia), multiple cerebral infarcts or chronic cerebral ischaemia

2 acute confusional states – usually of sudden onset in a patient who previously had normal higher cerebral function.

Chronic confusional state

This condition is characterised by gradual deterioration in intellectual, cognitive and memory functions of the brain with no clear disturbance of consciousness. Around 80% of cases are due to Alzheimer's disease.

Possible causes of chronic confusion include the following:

- Alzheimer's disease (80%)
- multi-infarct dementia – chronic cerebral ischaemia
- alcoholic dementia (including thiamine deficiency)
- subdural haematoma
- Wilson's disease
- Huntington's chorea
- syphilis.

Nervous system

CASE
54

With time the patient shows progressive impairment of short-term memory, visuospatial skills, language skills and social conduct. They become unable to cope with activities of daily living, and self-neglect becomes apparent. Unlike acute confusional states, there is no alteration in level of consciousness, impaired attention span or concentration, and a history of gradual deterioration over a period of months or years is the rule. Although patients have difficulty retaining new information and have poor short-term memory, their memory of past events – even back to recollections of childhood – is preserved and accurately recalled.

Acute confusional states

In these conditions there is often an associated reduction in the level of consciousness, and the time frame from normality to confusion is usually very short (hours or days).

Any condition that alters the normal functioning of the cells of the cerebral cortex can cause an acute confusional state. Common medical causes of acute confusion include the following:

1 Drugs:

- alcohol intoxication or withdrawal
- major and minor tranquillisers
- social drugs – ecstasy, narcotics, solvents and marijuana.

2 Major organ failure:

- cardiac failure
- hepatic encephalopathy
- renal failure.

3 Neurological disorders:

- epilepsy and post-ictal states
- encephalitis
- brain abscess
- cerebral vasculitis.

4 Raised intracranial pressure:

- meningitis
- cerebral tumour

CASE
54

- cerebrovascular events
- brain abscess.

5 Metabolic and endocrine causes:
- hyper- or hypoglycaemia
- hyper- or hyponatraemia
- hypoxia
- hypercapnia
- acidosis or alkalosis
- thyroid disease
- fever.

6 Trauma:
- head injury
- intracranial haematomas.

The priority is to rule out correctable raised intracranial pressure or infection, as either of these can lead to rapid deterioration and death.

The patient's ability to concentrate is impaired, and varying levels of depressed consciousness occur. Any association with pyrexia, meningeal irritation or raised white cell count should always suggest infection or subarachroid haemorrhage.

The presence of focal neurogical signs or papilloedema would suggest an intracranial mass or vascular lesion.

Clinical symptoms of cirrhosis would suggest the possibility of hepatic encephalopathy. However, one should always remain open-minded about other possible causes. For example, it is not uncommon for alcoholics to become intoxicated, fall over and sustain small fractures or intracranial bleeds. The acute confusional state associated with this is completely reversible by surgical drainage, provided that the diagnosis is considered and the confusional state is not simply attributed to alcohol excess.

Management

The management depends on the cause of the confusional state, and if possible should involve correction of the condition that has disrupted normal cerebral function.

When assessing a confused patient it is essential to take a history from a relative or close friend in order to establish the nature and duration of symptoms. Assessment of the patient involves determining whether or not there is an alteration in the level

Nervous system

CASE
54

of consciousness, assessing their mental state and assessing memory, language and cognitive function.

Assessing level of consciousness

Consciousness is the state of total awareness of oneself and one's environment. In acute confusional states there can be a depressed level of consciousness, which may fluctuate. It is important to document and monitor any change in the level of consciousness, as this may indicate progression of the condition or response to treatment.

The following simple grading system is commonly used:

Grade 5   Fully conscious and alert

Grade 4   Confused but able to answer simple questions

Grade 3   Unable to answer questions, but will obey commands
           (eg close your eyes, stick out your tongue)

Grade 2   Unresponsive to questions and commands, but gives semi-purposeful
           movement in response to pain

Grade 1   Reflex withdrawal movement to painful stimuli

Grade 0   Deeply unconscious and unresponsive even to pain

An alternative quantitative system is the Glasgow Coma Scale (see Table 12). This consists of a series of three major criteria, with scores given for each. The minimum score is 3 (indicating deeply unconscious) and the maximum is 15 (corresponding to fully conscious and alert).

Table 12 Glasgow Coma Scale

Eye opening	
None	1
Open in response to pain	2
Open in response to command	3
Spontaneous eye opening	4

continues . . .

CASE 54

Table 12 continued

Best motor response	
No movement	1
Abnormal extension with pain	2
Abnormal flexion with pain	3
Withdrawal response to pain	4
Localises to pain	5
Obeys commands to move	6
Best verbal response	
No speech	1
Incomprehensible	2
Inappropriate	3
Confused	4
Orientated	5

The mental state

Assessment of the mental state is used both in psychiatric assessment and to assess the intellectual and cognitive functions of patients who are confused. It can often help to discriminate between acute and chronic confusional states and psychiatric disorders in which language and memory are altered. Although in psychiatry a comprehensive assessment of the mental state requires prolonged and detailed questioning, for the purposes of confusional states due to medical disorders it is possible to perform an assessment relatively quickly using the Mini Mental State examination. Like the Glasgow Coma Scale, this uses a scoring system for a series of standard questions designed to assess memory, orientation, concentration, mental agility and language.

The Mini Mental State examination

For each * symbol that the patient answers correctly they score 1 point. The maximum possible score is 30, which indicates someone with a normal mental state who has good memory, mental agility and is well orientated. The lower the score the greater the degree of impairment of higher cerebral function.

Nervous system

CASE
54

Orientation questions

What is your name?*

Where do you live?*

What day is it today?*

Tell me today's date*, month* and year*.

What season is it?*

What is the name of this town/city?*

What county* and country* are we in?

Short-term memory

I want you to remember three objects (name three, eg toothbrush, boat, coat-hanger).

Ask the patient to repeat the words and score 1 for each word: toothbrush*, boat*, coat-hanger*. Repeat until all three remembered, allowing up to six attempts.

Attention and calculation

Ask the patient to serially subtract 7 from 100 and repeat the subtraction until they reach 65. Score 1 for each of the correct answers. Maximum score is 5 for 93*, 86*, 79*, 72*, and 65*.

Recall

'What were the three words I asked you to remember earlier?' Score 1 each for toothbrush*, boat* and coat-hanger*.

Language

Show the patient two simple objects and ask him or her to name them, eg pen* and watch*.

Ask the patient to repeat a nonsense phrase such as 'No ifs, ands or buts'*.

Ask the patient to read a statement and do as it says, eg 'lift your left hand above your head'. Score if they perform the task*.

Ask the patient to write down a short simple sentence which you dictate, eg 'I walk my dog every day'*.

Ask the patient to perform a series of simple tasks, eg 'Take this piece of paper off the desk*, fold it in half* and place it on the floor'*.

Ask the patient to copy a drawing (eg two pentagons which have five sides and overlap)*.

Nervous system

CASE
54

CASE 55

Depression

Depression can cause a variety of symptoms and must be considered at history-taking stations where patients describe tiredness, generalised pain or alteration of memory. It is also important at OSCE stations concerned with drug overdose or assessment of the mental state.

Definition and classification

Depression is an alteration in mood associated with feelings of sadness, worthlessness and lack of motivation or hope.

Depression can be part of a bipolar mood disorder in which the patient swings between depression and mania, or it may be a unipolar disorder associated with feelings of depression only. It can also be either reactive (resulting from some life event, eg illness or bereavement) or endogenous (where there is no known underlying cause).

Clinical features

Everyone feels sad or 'down in the dumps' at some times in their life, but when such feelings become pervasive and interfere with an individual's normal functioning or ability to cope with activities of daily living, then clinical depression is said to be present. Women are more commonly affected with depressive illness, and the prevalence in divorced or separated individuals is approximately three times higher than that in single or married people.

Depression affects the mood, thinking, speech and the drive or energy of the individual, and it can cause subjective physical symptoms, especially lack of energy, fatigue, generalised muscle and joint pains, headache, weight loss and alterations in short-term memory and cognitive function. In its most extreme form it can cause major disability and result in attempts at self-harm or suicide.

Anxiety, panic attacks or obsessional behaviour are common associated abnormalities, and sometimes phobias can occur.

A classic sleep pattern disturbance characterised by early-morning wakening is common, with the patient spontaneously awakening at 4 to 6 am and unable to get

Nervous system

CASE
55

back to sleep. Often the feeling of depression is most severe in the early morning, with ideas of suicide and worthlessness prominent.

Frequently the patient may display feelings of guilt or a sense of bodily disease. Their ability to remember, concentrate and take in new information is adversely affected, which may raise the suspicion of dementia or an organic brain disorder.

Loss of appetite with associated weight loss is common, and loss of libido frequently occurs.

Investigations

Physical disorders that can cause many of the physical symptoms must be ruled out. Anaemia, hypothyroidism and organic brain syndromes can be assessed by full blood picture, thyroid function tests and CT or MRI scans of the brain.

Treatment

Careful history taking is essential to try to identify whether the mood disorder is a reactive depression due to some remediable stress or life event. Psychotherapy or counselling can be extremely helpful for depression.

The mood disorder can be treated with antidepressant medication. The main groups of drugs used are as follows:

1. Tricyclic antidepressants (eg amitriptyline). It can take up to three or four weeks before the onset of maximum effect of these drugs is apparent. They may also cause side effects such as nausea, blurring of vision or cardiac arrhythmias.

2. Serotonin re-uptake inhibitors (eg fluoxetine, sertraline). These improve the mood by increasing the levels of serotonin (5-hydroxytryptamine) in the brain.

In severe or drug-resistant cases, electroconvulsive therapy (ECT) is used. This form of therapy should only be used in specialist psychiatric centres, after a careful assessment of the patient has been made and informed consent given for the procedure.

Most patients who are treated for depression make a good recovery (within 6–9 months), but 25–30% will have a recurrence of their mood disorder within one year, and 75% within a 10-year period.

Nervous system

CASE
55

CASE 56

Overdose (self-poisoning)

This is one of the commonest reasons why young people (under 35 years of age) are admitted to acute medical units, and students are expected to be able to manage the common forms of overdose and know the general principles of management.

Definition

Overdose is the taking of poisons or drugs in excessive dosage to cause self-harm or as a 'cry-for-help' gesture, often associated with mental depression or as a result of psychological pressure or stress.

Causes

Acute overdose usually involves more than one drug, and alcohol is commonly the second agent in this situation. The patient who is depressed or psychologically disturbed may drink alcohol and then ingest a quantity of medication that has been prescribed or bought over the counter.

The following drugs are commonly used:

- paracetamol
- antidepressants
- minor tranquillisers
- hypnotic drugs (sleeping pills)
- non-steroidal anti-inflammatory drugs.

Clinical features

The patient is often intoxicated with alcohol, and if sleeping pills or tranquillisers have been taken he or she will have a reduced level of consciousness. The other clinical features and the management will depend on the type and quantity of substance that has been ingested.

In all cases, once the type of drug has been determined, information should be obtained from the nearest poisons information centre to determine what clinical

Nervous system

CASE 56

features may develop, the lethal dose or blood level, what treatment should be administered and, in particular, what antidote (if any) can be used.

If the drug has not been identified, a serum sample should be sent for an urgent toxicology screen to look for levels of the following:

- ethanol
- methanol
- theophylline
- amphetamine
- digoxin
- paracetamol
- lithium
- aspirin
- paraquat
- tricyclic antidepressant.

Investigations

In addition to toxicology screening, the following investigations are needed:

1 biochemical profile – to ensure that there is normal fluid and electrolyte balance and renal function
2 blood glucose – to ensure that the patient has not injected insulin (hypoglycaemia) or developed hyperglycaemia as a result of salicylate poisoning
3 liver function tests should be performed, particularly in patients who have taken paracetamol
4 patients who have overdosed with tricyclic antidepressants or amphetamines must undergo ECG monitoring, as they may develop life-threatening arrhythmias.

Treatment

Most patients require only supportive care, and after 24–48 hours they will have fully recovered, having metabolised and/or excreted the bulk of the drugs ingested. For patients who are deeply unconscious or who have respiratory depression, intensive care and respiratory support may be necessary in the early stages. If hypotension

develops, intravenous fluids are used to maintain the systolic blood pressure at
> 90 mmHg so that renal perfusion is preserved.

Specific antidotes should be used where indicated (some of the more commonly used
antidotes are listed in Table 13). Otherwise action can be taken to try to reduce
absorption of the poison or ingested drug by administering activated charcoal by
mouth or, if the ingested material is non-corrosive and there is no risk of aspiration,
inducing vomiting or performing gastric lavage to empty the stomach of its contents.

Table 13 Antidotes used in cases of poisoning

Poison	Antidote
Paracetamol	N-acetylcysteine
Warfarin	Vitamin K
Digoxin	Digoxin-specific antibody fragments
Benzodiazepine	Flumazenil
Heroin/morphine	Naloxone

Once the patient is conscious and capable of understanding, their mental state should
be assessed and they should be asked why the overdose was taken. In particular,
they should be asked if they were trying to take their own life. If there is any
suspicion that this event was a deliberate suicide attempt, the patient must receive
expert psychiatric assessment before they can be discharged.

If the overdose was a 'cry-for-help' gesture, the patient should be given the
opportunity to speak to a psychiatrist either before discharge or as an outpatient
(provided that they are not at risk of another overdose).

Nervous system

CASE
56

CASE 57

Cranial nerve examination

This clinical station is often used in the OSCE, either to assess the competence of the student in systematically examining all of the cranial nerves in a short period of time, or to assess their ability to identify a specific cranial nerve palsy and discuss the most common causes. The examination of each cranial nerve and the commonest causes of nerve damage are discussed below.

I Olfactory nerve

Ask the patient about smell and taste. Remember that the tongue can only detect four tastes – all other flavours are smelt. For this reason, patients with damage to the olfactory nerve cannot taste their food properly.

Examine each nostril individually while the other nostril is occluded. Use odour bottles containing camphor, menthol and ammonia salts. With their eyes closed, ask the patient to identify each smell.

Anosmia is the complete loss of a sense of smell, and may occur as a result of mechanical occlusion of a nasal passage by a foreign body or tumour, or damage to the first cranial nerve on the same side due to tumours of the nasal passage, sinuses or frontal lobes infiltrating the nerve.

II Optic nerve

Ask the patient whether they have noticed any change in their vision.

Test their visual acuity. Increasing degrees of visual impairment are roughly assessed as inability to read small newsprint, to read headlines, to count fingers accurately, to see hand movement, and to perceive light. A more accurate assessment of acuity can be achieved using a Snellen chart.

Test their visual fields. These are assessed clinically by confrontation (see Case 64) and more precisely by perimetry. Defects in visual fields are discussed on page 188.

Test the direct and consensual light reflex. The afferent fibres for the light reflex are carried in the optic nerve, and the efferent fibres are carried in the oculomotor nerve. Therefore, if a patient has left optic nerve damage there will be blindness in the left eye together with loss of the direct reflex in the left eye and no consensual reflex in

CASE
57

the right eye, but a normal light reflex in the right eye with a normal consensual reflex in the left eye.

III Oculomotor nerve, IV Trochlear nerve and VI Abducens nerve

These three nerves are usually tested together, as they are responsible for the innervation of the extraocular muscles. The muscles that they serve are easily remembered by the formula LR6(SO4)3, where:

LR = lateral rectus ie sixth cranial nerve (6)

SO = superior oblique ie fourth cranial nerve (4)

( )3 = all others ie oculomotor motor or third nerve (3).

- Paralysis of III – results in the unopposed action of lateral rectus and superior oblique muscles, and the eye on the affected side is held looking 'down and out'
- Paralysis of IV – the eye on the affected side is unable to look down and ~~outwards~~ inwards
- Paralysis of VI – results in inability to abduct the eye on the affected side, and the patient experiences double vision on looking towards that side.

The oculomotor nerve also carries fibres which innervate the levator palpebrae superioris muscle of the upper eyelid and the nerve fibres responsible for pupillary constriction. Third nerve palsy is therefore also associated with ptosis and dilatation of the pupil.

This nerve also arises from its cranial nerve nucleus in the floor of the aqueduct of Sylvius and runs a long course within the cranium. During its course it bends over the tentorium cerebelli. Any cause of raised intracranial pressure can result in initial irritation of the nerve, causing pupillary constriction on the affected side and, if the pressure increases further, paralysis of the nerve, which results in a fixed dilated pupil, ptosis and loss of function of the extraocular muscles it supplies.

Nervous system

CASE
57

V Trigeminal nerve

This nerve has sensory and motor functions, and it has three divisions:

1 ophthalmic – sensory areas of conjunctiva, forehead, upper eyelid and inside of the nose

2 maxillary – sensory to the cheek, front of the temple, side of the nose, upper lip and teeth

3 mandibular – carries sensory fibres to the skin over the lower jaw and lip, and motor fibres which innervate the muscles of mastication (masseter and pterygoids).

Damage to this nerve or to one of its divisions results in sensory loss of the affected area and/or paralysis of the muscles.

It should also be remembered that the sensory representation at the nerve nucleus is in a muzzle distribution. If lesions of the elongated nucleus in the midbrain occur in the upper region, they result in loss of sensation of the skin on the nose, while damage further down causes a widening area of sensory loss in a concentric fashion across the face.

VII Facial nerve

The facial nerve supplies the muscles of facial expression and carries taste fibres to the anterior two-thirds of the tongue from the chorda tympani. The muscles of facial expression of the forehead are represented on both cerebral cortices, and therefore the pattern of muscle weakness which is present can easily allow differentiation between upper and lower motor neurone lesions. In upper motor neurone lesions, which may commonly occur as a result of a stroke, there is paralysis of the muscles on the lower part of the face on the affected side but the patient is still able to raise their eyebrow and close their eye tightly. In a lower motor neurone seventh nerve palsy, which can occur as a result of Bell's palsy, a parotid tumour or damage to the nerve as it passes through the parotid gland, there is complete paralysis of all the muscles of facial expression on the affected side, including those of the forehead and orbicularis oculi muscle.

VIII Auditory nerve

Damage to this nerve can be caused by tumours of the brain, acoustic neuromas or invasion of the nerve by tumour spreading from the auditory canal. It results in deafness, and must be differentiated from other causes of impaired hearing (see page 190).

CASE 57

IX Glossopharyngeal nerve, X Vagus nerve and XI Accessory nerve

These nerves arise from elongated nuclei in the floor of the fourth ventricle and several roots along the lateral aspect of the medulla. Brainstem infarcts, haemorrhage or tumours can result in nerve damage.

The glossopharyngeal nerve innervates the muscles of the pharynx and soft palate and carries taste sensory fibres to the posterior third of the tongue. The vagus nerve carries the main parasympathetic fibres to the major organs of the thorax and abdomen. It also supplies the muscles of the pharynx and soft palate. Damage to either of these nerves results in loss of the gag reflex and failure of elevation of the soft palate when the patient is asked to phonate.

The accessory nerve supplies motor fibres to the accessory muscles of respiration (the sternomastoid and the upper fibres of the trapezius). Paralysis results in weakness of these muscles and an inability to shrug the shoulder on the affected side or to contract the sternomastoid against resistance.

XII Hypoglossal nerve

This nerve supplies the hypoglossal muscles, which are used to protrude the tongue. Because the muscles are attached to the mandible and cross as they run posteriorly to the underside of the tongue, paralysis of one hypoglossal nerve will result in deviation of the tongue towards the affected side when the patient is asked to stick out their tongue.

Nervous system

CASE
57

CASE 58

Power, tone, co-ordination and reflexes

This clinical station can be used to assess the student's ability to examine the motor system of the upper and/or lower limbs, which may simply involve performing the examination on a normal volunteer. It may also be used to assess the student's ability to detect abnormal signs in patients with neurological disorders. Patients with any of the following conditions may commonly be encountered:

1 hemiplegia or hemiparesis

2 Parkinson's disease

3 multiple sclerosis

4 motor neurone disease.

The specific features of these individual disorders are discussed in Cases 60 and 62.

Approach to the examination of power, tone and reflexes

If you are asked to examine the limbs and assess power, tone and reflexes, always start by making a general inspection and comment on the following:

1 **Posture.** Is a limb held in an abnormal position, such as a flexion deformity resulting from a contracture?

2 **Muscle wasting.** Do the limbs appear symmetrical with regard to size, shape and muscle bulk? Muscle wasting will occur in primary muscle disorders such as muscular dystrophy, or if there are lower motor neurone lesions.

3 **Abnormal movement.** Is there evidence of any involuntary movement of the whole limb or limbs? On inspection of individual limbs, is there any evidence of fasciculation of muscle fibres?

Next perform a physical examination and assess tone, power and co-ordination.

CASE 58

Tone

This is the state of reflex partial contraction that all muscle groups normally exhibit. Any interruption of the impulses coming to muscle fibres via the lower motor neurone that supplies them will result in loss of this partial contraction, with hypotonia and subsequent wasting will result.

If damage occurs to the upper motor neurone of the nerve pathway to muscle fibres, the spinal reflex will be increased, with resulting hypertonia of the muscle.

To test tone, first ask the patient if they have any pain or discomfort in the limbs that you are about to examine. Ask them to relax their limbs totally, and inform them that you are going to gently move them through a range of movements.

While gently flexing and extending the limb, assess whether or not the tone of the muscles around each joint is normal, increased or decreased, and compare sides. When examining the lower limbs it is important to test for clonus. This is performed with the patient's leg semi-flexed at the knee joint. Ensuring that the foot and muscles around the ankle joint are relaxed, gently move the patient's foot up and down. Then suddenly dorsiflex and slightly evert the foot, and hold it in this position for several seconds. If there is increased tone in the calf muscles, the foot will uncontrollably flex and relax repeatedly. Clonus is present if more than five reflex contractions occur.

Power

If you are asked to test power in the upper or lower limbs, remember to test all of the muscle groups, including the small muscles of the hands and feet. Demonstrate a considerate method of testing which does not cause pain or discomfort to the patient, and let the examiner observe that you are testing the strength of each muscle group against resistance and, in patients with muscle weakness, with gravity eliminated. Use the Medical Research Council grading system to describe the power (see Table 14).

It is most important that you test and compare the strength of muscle groups on both sides of the body. For example, test the muscles of abduction of the left shoulder joint followed by those of the right shoulder joint.

To eliminate the force of gravity, test power with the limb held in a position horizontal to the ground so that muscle contraction in this plane will only have to overcome the resistance caused by the weight of the limb.

Develop a sequence of testing power in all limbs that is comfortable both for the patient and for yourself, and that assesses all of the major muscle groups.

Nervous system

CASE
58

Table 14 Medical Research Council grading system for muscle power

Grade 5	Normal – full strength
Grade 4	Reduced power, but able to move against gravity and resistance
Grade 3	Capable of movement against gravity, but unable to move against any further resistance
Grade 2	Unable to move against the force of gravity, but capable of movement when gravity is eliminated
Grade 1	Muscle contraction, but no movement of the limb even when gravity is eliminated
Grade 0	No muscle contraction when the patient attempts to move

Co-ordination

This is the ability to perform accurate movements. It requires normal functioning of the cerebellum and posterior columns of the spinal cord. Disorders of cerebellar function or proprioception result in unco-ordinated, clumsy movements. However, it must be remembered that if there is muscle weakness of a limb this may give the appearance of lack of co-ordination. It is vital therefore that before any decision about co-ordination is reached, muscle power is carefully assessed.

Finger–nose test

This test is used to examine co-ordination of the upper limbs. With your index finger held 2–3 feet away from the patient's face, ask them to move their right index finger quickly to touch your finger and then the tip of their own nose repeatedly. While they are performing this action, move your finger up and down slightly and observe how accurately they are adjusting their movements so that they find the target for which they are aiming. Ask them to repeat the test using their left hand.

The abnormalities that you are trying to detect and which are characteristic of cerebellar dysfunction on the ipsilateral (same) side of the body are intention tremor, dysmetria (past-pointing) and ataxia.

Intention tremor

Each time the patient's finger moves towards your finger, there is an increasing magnitude of oscillation of their hand.

CASE
58

Dysmetria (past-pointing)

The patient is unable to accurately stop their finger at the exact position of your finger. They either strike your finger with enough force to push it backwards, or miss your finger completely and end each action with their finger well beyond yours.

Ataxia

The path of movement of the patient's hand between their own nose and your object finger is not straight. This is because they are incapable of finely controlling the accessory agonist and antagonist muscles needed for flowing accurate movement. This function can also be assessed by asking the patient to perform a task that requires alternating movements.

Ask the patient to repeatedly move the fingers of each hand as if they are playing the piano, but in a sequence starting each time with the little finger. Alternatively, ask the patient to repeatedly pronate and supinate their hand, each time tapping the palm and dorsum of one hand on the palm of their other hand. If they are incapable of performing either or both of these tests with an accurate, flowing and co-ordinated movement, this indicates an abnormality of the extrapyramidal system (usually an ipsilateral cerebellar disorder). The unco-ordinated movements are known as dysdiadochokinesia.

Heel–shin test

This is used to assess co-ordination of the lower limbs. The test is performed with the patient lying on a bed or examination couch with both lower legs fully exposed. The patient is asked to accurately place the heel of one foot on the shin bone of their other leg just below the knee, and then to carefully run the heel down the shin bone to the ankle, lift the heel off and replace it in position just below the knee again. When they have repeated the movement a few times they should be asked to perform the test again using the heel of the other foot. Patients with ataxia of the legs cannot perform these movements in a co-ordinated flowing manner.

Patients who have problems with ataxia, loss of co-ordination or proprioception will display abnormalities of gait, and this should be assessed. When they walk they often have a wide, sometimes stamping gait. They may tend to walk or fall over to one side, and they may have difficulty turning around. When assessing gait it is vitally important that you accompany the patient and ensure that they do not fall over or injure themselves.

Nervous system

CASE
58

Romberg's test

Ask the patient to stand facing you with their feet approximately six inches apart and their eyes open. Observe how steady they are for a few seconds, and then ask them to close their eyes. Again observe the patient's ability to maintain their equilibrium when they lose the visual cues for position. If they become unsteady or show a tendency to fall, this is a positive Romberg's sign and indicates a disorder of proprioception.

Reflexes

This is a very discriminating test of a student's clinical ability, and it is frequently used in OSCEs. It tests not only the student's skill in using a tendon hammer, but also their ability to get the patient to relax fully and co-operate with the testing procedure, and to perform a test which involves striking the patient without causing pain or discomfort. It can also be used to assess the student's knowledge of anatomy, pathology and neurology. When testing reflexes it is important that the patient is relaxed and comfortably positioned and that the limbs being examined are fully exposed. The proper use of the tendon hammer is extremely important – in fact, this piece of equipment is badly named because the one thing that you must never do is use it to hammer a tendon.

The object of the test is to deliver an identical force to tendons that are being held under tension. The force causes a transient stretching of the attached muscle and produces a reflex arc carried by sensory afferent and motor efferent neurones, resulting in muscle contraction. Comparing the force of contraction is the aim of the test. If the equipment is used as a hammer, it is impossible to deliver an identical force with each test. This can only be achieved by allowing the force of gravity to drop the hammer each time from a constant distance to strike the tendon. This ensures that the force delivered to the tendon is always constant and is a function of the weight of the hammer, the force of gravity and the distance that the hammer has fallen – all of which are or can be kept constant. Any variation in reflex contraction between the two sides will be due to a change in the reflex arc and not due to variation in the force that was applied to the tendon.

Test all reflexes while the patient has the limb completely relaxed, but you must ensure that the tendon is held under some degree of tension so that when it is struck it will stretch the attached muscle.

During the test, let the examiner know that you are observing the muscle as well as feeling or watching the degree of movement of the limb.

CASE
58

Test all reflexes and familiarise yourself with the spinal level of the reflex arc for each of them:

Reflex	Spinal level
Biceps	C5 C6
Triceps	C6 C7 C8
Supinator	C6 C7
Hoffmann's	C7 C8
Knee	L2 L3 L4
Ankle	S1 S2

Remember to test for finger jerks and Hoffmann's reflex. The latter is performed by supporting the middle phalanx of the patient's middle finger and quickly flicking the distal phalanx downwards with your thumb. A positive Hoffmann's reflex occurs when the patient's thumb reflexly flexes, and is a sign of hyper-reflexia or increased tone in the affected limb.

Plantar reflex (Babinski's sign)

This should be performed using a pointed though not sharp object, such as the end of an orange stick or key. Expose the foot and ensure that the toes are relaxed. Run the pointed implement along the lateral aspect of the plantar surface of the foot and then medially across the skin over the heads of the metatarsals. Babinski's sign is positive if dorsiflexion of the big toe occurs. It is a sign of an upper motor neurone lesion.

Finally, remember that if you are having difficulty eliciting reflexes you should use reinforcement: ask the patient to perform a purposeful movement, such as clenching their teeth or interlocking the fingers of both hands and then pulling the hands apart while keeping the fingers interlocked just before and during your attempt.

Nervous system

CASE
58

CASE 59

Sensory examination

Testing sensation in the limbs is a common OSCE station. It can be used to assess the student's technique and systematic approach with a normal subject, or to determine whether the student can detect and interpret abnormal findings in a real patient.

Sensory modalities to be tested include the following:

1   pain – pinprick

2   temperature – hot/cold

3   touch – light touch

4   vibration and proprioception

5   recognition of shapes and sizes.

A knowledge of the paths of the sensory tracts in the spinal cord and brain is essential in order to interpret clinical findings (see Fig 3).

Fig 3 Sensory and motor tracts of spinal cord.

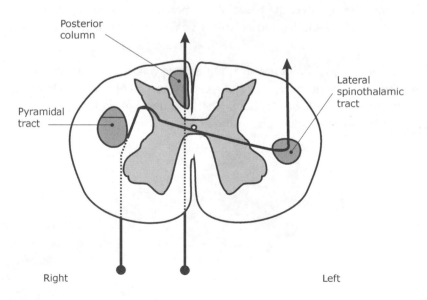

Pain

Pain sensory neurones enter the cord via the dorsal root, cross immediately to the lateral spinothalamic tract on the opposite side and then ascend to the thalamus. Testing is performed using sharp and blunt implements. Damage to these neurones results in hypoalgesia, analgesia or possibly hyperalgesia. Like temperature sensory neurones, pain fibres cross the cord at the level at which they enter. Therefore, damage to the cord results in loss of pain sensation on the contralateral side of the body below the level of the lesion. Damage to the posterior root of the nerve or to the peripheral nerve results in loss of sensation at and below the level of damage, on the same side.

Temperature

This can be tested using two test tubes or glass flasks, one containing hot and one containing cold liquid. The patient is asked to close their eyes and identify which container is touching their skin. The temperature sensory neurones are also carried in the lateral spinothalamic tracts, and the distribution of loss is identical to that which occurs for pain.

Touch

Light touch sensation is tested using a wisp of cotton wool. The patient is asked to close their eyes and say 'yes' when their skin is lightly brushed with the cotton wool. The neurones that carry light touch sensation enter via the posterior nerve root, cross the cord and ascend to the thalamus with half in the lateral spinothalamic tract and half in the anterior spinothalamic tract. Damage to the cord in this region results in loss of touch sensation below this level on the contralateral side.

By testing the limbs in a systematic fashion it is possible to:

1 identify a cord lesion – loss of sensation in the distribution of a dermatome
2 identify damage to the peripheral nerve of the posterior root – 'glove or stocking' sensory loss. This is the type of sensory loss that is more commonly encountered in clinical examinations (See Case 61).

Vibration and proprioception

Vibration sensation is tested using a large tuning fork. Strike the prongs and place the non-vibrating end against a bony prominence such as the tibial tubercle or medial malleolus. Ask the patient if they can detect the vibration of the fork. If they cannot, move progressively proximally until the sensation is detected.

Nervous system

CASE
59

Proprioception (joint-position sensation) is tested in the lower limbs by exposing the feet and toes. Ask the patient to close their eyes and then instruct them to determine the position of their big toe while you carefully move the distal phalanx up or down. In the upper limbs a similar test can be performed using the thumbs, or you can ask the patient to close their eyes while you move their arm, and then ask them to grasp the thumb of the arm that has been moved with their other hand. Normal joint-position sensation is essential for the patient to determine the position of their limb accurately without a visual cue.

Both vibration and proprioception sensory neurones ascend on the same side as they enter, and are carried in the posterior columns of the cord. Damage to the cord in this region therefore results in loss of proprioception and vibration sense on the same side as the damage.

From the above account it is clear that hemisection of the spinal cord (ie unilateral damage to the cord) will result in loss of pain and temperature sensation on the opposite side and loss of vibration and proprioception on the same side. Damage to the pyramidal tracts, which carry motor function, will result in loss of power with the characteristics of an upper motor neurone lesion below the level of the damage on the same side. This combination of neurological features is known as Brown-Séquard's syndrome.

Recognition of shapes and sizes

The part of the brain that is responsible for tactile discrimination of size and shape is the parietal lobe. Lesions of this area result in the inability to recognise objects by touch alone (astereognosis). Because the touch sensory fibres cross the cord on entry, lesions of the left parietal lobe cause astereognosis when objects are placed in the right hand, and vice versa.

Another feature of parietal lobe damage is loss of two-point discrimination, which can be tested using a pair of dividers. A patient with a parietal lobe lesion is unable to discern the fact that the two points of a pair of dividers, widely spaced, which are touching the skin of a limb on the opposite side of the body are two separate points of contact. Instead, the stimulus is felt as a single point. This sensory deficit can also be detected by asking the patient, with their eyes closed, to identify numbers that are 'written' on the palm of their hand with a blunt object or your fingertip. However, these abnormalities should only be looked for in a patient with otherwise normal sensation in the limbs.

CASE 59

CASE 60

Parkinsonism

There are many patients in the community with parkinsonism who are willing to be used for medical examination purposes. This condition is ideal for use as a clinical station to assess the student's approach to neurological examination and detection of abnormalities.

Definition

Parkinsonism is an abnormality of extrapyramidal function due to cell loss and dopamine deficiency in the extrapyramidal nuclei, resulting in disturbances of posture and movement.

? Causes

These include the following:

1 Idiopathic (Parkinson's disease)

2 Secondary (parkinsonism)

- cerebral ischaemia
- post-encephalitic
- heavy metal poisoning (eg manganese)
- carbon monoxide poisoning.

3 Drugs:

- phenothiazines (chlorpromazine)
- benzamides (metoclopramide)
- designer hallucinogenic drugs (MPTP).

Nervous system

CASE
60

Clinical features

The triad of rigidity, tremor and bradykinesia is the hallmark of this condition, although the presence and severity of these signs can vary from one patient to another.

In the early stages the patient may only display general slowing down, an expressionless face and reduced accessory movement (eg they stop swinging their arms while walking). Later a tremor develops, which may initially be unilateral. Classically the tremor is of a 'pill-rolling' nature (six cycles per second). As the disease progresses, muscle rigidity, a shuffling gait and problems with initiating new movements can develop. On examination, the classic clinical signs are increased tone superimposed on the tremor (cogwheel rigidity) and a positive glabellar tap. Repeated tapping on the glabella (the area of skin between the eyes) results in the patient involuntarily blinking with each tap, whereas normal individuals will stop blinking after two or three taps. Micrographia may also occur, and the handwriting becomes small even during the writing of a single sentence.

In some patients an autonomic neuropathy may develop (Shy-Drager syndrome), with postural hypotension as a prominent feature.

Treatment

Initially, supportive measures are used after assessment by occupational therapists and physiotherapists in an effort to maintain mobility and allow the patient to function normally for as long as possible.

Antiparkinsonian drugs

1. L-Dopa is the mainstay of treatment. This replaces the deficiency and can be used in conjuction with a decarboxylase inhibitor to give an increased dose response by reducing the metabolism of the drug.

2. Selegiline, a type B monoamine oxidase inhibitor, may be useful.

3. Dopamine agonists (eg lisuride or bromocriptine) are used, usually in the latter stages of the disease.

4. Anticholinergic drugs (eg benzhexol or orphenadrine) are used to treat the tremor. However, side effects are common with this group of drugs, which may not be tolerated, especially in elderly patients.

CASE
60

ʟ-Dopa is usually introduced at an early stage and the dose gradually increased. However, over a period of time the duration of effect may decrease and patients may experience an 'on-off' effect. This can be corrected by giving smaller doses more frequently, or by administering apomorphine by subcutaneous injection if the on-off effect is very troublesome.

The prognosis of Parkinson's disease is usually one of gradual progression, with a life expectancy of approximately 15 years from diagnosis.

Nervous system

CASE
60

CASE 61

Peripheral neuropathy

Peripheral neuropathy can affect nerves that carry power and/or sensory fibres. However, the condition is most commonly encountered at clinical examination stations, where students are usually asked to examine the sensation in either the upper or lower limbs.

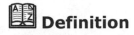 Definition

Peripheral neuropathy is a disorder of one or more peripheral nerves, resulting in impaired sensation in that area from which sensory afferent fibres arise that are carried by the nerves, and/or loss of power in the muscles supplied by lower motor neurones carried by the nerves.

? Causes

There are two ways in which peripheral nerve damage can occur:

1 loss of the myelin sheath

2 neuronal death (axonal damage).

One or both of these mechanisms can result from any of the following:

- toxins (eg alcohol, heavy metal poisoning)
- deficiency states, especially deficiency of vitamin B_{12} or B_6
- vascular disease, especially as a microvascular complication of diabetes mellitus or due to vasculitis affecting the blood supply to the nerves.

Clinical features

The nerves that have the longest axons are most susceptible to damage, and therefore the symptoms and signs usually affect the distal regions of the limbs first (ie the toes and fingers) and then move proximally as the condition progresses.

Nervous system

CASE 61

If the condition is affecting a predominantly motor nerve, the symptoms and signs are of weakness of the small muscles of the feet and hands. More commonly, however, sensory symptoms are experienced by the patient as the long nerves carry many sensory fibres, and the patient complains of 'pins and needles' or numbness of the toes and feet which may later also affect the fingers and hands in a 'glove and stocking' distribution. On examination there is loss of sensation with regard to light touch and pinprick, which starts at the distal point of the affected limb and extends in a proximal direction. Usually a relatively clear line of demarcation can be determined between the areas of sensory loss and normal sensation.

On testing the power of the small intrinsic muscles of the hands or feet, evidence of muscle weakness is found if the affected nerve has a motor function.

Investigations

These aim to:

1 confirm that the peripheral nerve function is abnormal

2 determine the nature of the underlying cause.

Nerve conduction studies are used to assess the rate of transmission of electrical stimuli along peripheral nerves, and can differentiate between peripheral neuropathy and myopathy as a cause of muscle weakness in the hands or feet.

A routine full blood picture may show evidence of a macrocytic hyperchromic anaemia, indicating vitamin B_{12} or folate deficiency. A serum vitamin B_{12} assay could confirm that this deficiency state exists as a possible cause.

The clinical history is usually sufficient to determine whether excessive alcohol consumption or diabetes mellitus are likely causes, while a rheumatoid factor assay or a positive pANCA test might indicate vasculitis as the likely cause.

Treatment

This depends on the underlying cause. If the condition is due to vitamin B_{12} or B_6 deficiency, replacement therapy can reverse the damage and complete recovery is possible. Similarly, if it is the result of excess alcohol consumption, the symptoms are likely to improve if the patient abstains from alcohol.

Vasculitis can be treated with steroids, which often improve or reverse the symptoms if treatment is given at an early stage (ie before axonal destruction occurs). For patients with diabetes, strict control of blood sugar levels is the best means of preventing further deterioration in symptoms.

Nervous system

CASE
61

CASE 62

Paraparesis and multiple sclerosis

Multiple sclerosis is a relatively common chronic neurological disorder, and it can readily be used in clinical OSCE stations to test the student's ability to elicit and interpret abnormal clinical signs. It is also one of the commoner causes of paraparesis, and for this reason the two conditions are here considered together.

Paraparesis

Definition

Paraparesis is a weakness of the lower limbs, and can be either a **flaccid paraparesis** (weakness with reduced tone due to bilateral lower motor neurone lesions) or, more commonly, a **spastic paraparesis** (weakness with increased tone due to a lesion or lesions in the spinal cord causing bilateral upper motor neurone weakness).

? Causes

There are many causes of paraparesis, but the most common ones are trauma resulting in spinal cord damage below the level of the cervical cord, and multiple sclerosis resulting in the development of areas of demyelination in the cord.

The main causes can be summarised as follows:

- trauma
- multiple sclerosis
- spinal cord compression
- motor neurone disease
- subacute combined degeneration of the cord
- syringomyelia
- spinal cord ischaemia
- myelitis (inflammatory lesions affecting the cord).

CASE 62

Multiple sclerosis

Definition

Multiple sclerosis is a demyelinating disorder of unknown aetiology that causes lesions in the brain and/or spinal cord which result in both upper and lower motor neurone lesions and sensory nerve damage.

Clinical features

Multiple sclerosis can affect any age group, but most often has an onset between the ages of 20 and 40 years. Its incidence is the same in both sexes. It may present initially as an episode of visual disturbance due to retrobulbar neuritis, which may resolve completely. The disease is usually characterised by episodes of neurological symptoms in a pattern of relapses and remissions. The common symptoms are as follows:

- **Muscle weakness.** This usually affects the lower limbs initially. Often the patient may start to fall or trip over their own feet due to foot drop on one or both sides. With each relapse the degree of weakness gets progressively worse.

- **Urinary symptoms.** With the development of demyelinating plaques in the region of the cord that supplies innervation to the bladder, the patient may develop urgency, frequency or incontinence. These symptoms usually only develop in association with bilateral leg weakness.

- **Unsteadiness.** Involvement of the cerebellum or the posterior columns of the spinal cord can result in ataxia, lack of co-ordination of movement and unsteadiness, with a positive Romberg's test.

- **Eye signs.** Involvement of the optic nerve or optic pathway can result in visual impairment, with central or arcuate scotomas or tunnel vision. Damage to the optic nerve can be seen on fundoscopy as temporal pallor of the optic nerve head in the early stages, or as optic atrophy later on (see page 204). If the nerve tracts that control conjugate eye movements (medial longitudinal fasciculus) are involved, the patient may develop double vision (diplopia), and on examination there is loss of conjugate eye movements, when the eyes move independently of one another. Involvement of the cerebellum will cause nystagmus, which can be horizontal, vertical or rotatory.

- **Spastic paraparesis.** If demyelination occurs in the cord and affects the motor neurones, a spastic paraparesis may develop below the level of the lesions. This is characterised by weakness of the lower limbs that is

Nervous system

CASE
62

associated with increased tone, normal muscle bulk, increased reflexes and an extensor plantar reflex. Other features of increased tone may be demonstrated, such as patellar or ankle clonus.

In multiple sclerosis, sensory symptoms and signs often occur due to demyelination affecting the neurones in the spinothalamic tracts or posterior columns of the cord.

Patients may complain of paraesthesia or numbness, and on examination objective sensory loss may be found, the nature of which will depend on precisely which sensory neurones are affected.

Demyelination can affect any part of the central or peripheral nervous system. If the frontal lobes are involved, the patient may display a personality change or their behaviour may become disinhibited and their mood euphoric.

Investigations

The best imaging method is MRI scanning, which shows demyelinating plaques in the brain and/or spinal cord.

Visual-evoked response testing can be used to demonstrate slowing of nerve conduction velocity in the neurones of the visual pathway. Lumbar puncture with analysis of the cerebrospinal fluid may reveal a slight increase in mononuclear cells. Normal or slightly increased levels of protein and oligoclonal antibodies may be detected.

Treatment

Many patients with mild disease require no therapy. Acute relapses can be treated with steroids (prednisolone), either alone or together with cytotoxic drugs (eg azathioprine as a steroid-sparing agent).

Interferon is used in some patients to reduce the frequency and/or severity of relapse, but this drug treatment is not beneficial in all cases, is expensive and is not without side effects. Its effectiveness is still being studied in large multicentre clinical trials.

Nervous system

CASE
62

Prognosis

Multiple sclerosis is a chronic disorder with a variable and unpredictable course in any individual patient. Overall, however, in a population of patients with the disorder, after 20 years around 20% of individuals would be asymptomatic or have minimal disability, 60% would have significant disability due to neurological disease and 20% would have died (usually as a result of infection of the respiratory system, or septicaemia complicating respiratory or renal infection).

Nervous system

CASE
62

CASE 63

Cerebellar disease

It is very easy for an actor or examiner to simulate the clinical features of cerebellar disease, and therefore this condition is often used in a clinical examination station.

Definition

Cerebellar disease refers to any condition that affects the ability of the cerebellum to control and co-ordinate motor function and movement.

Causes

A wide variety of underlying medical conditions can affect the cerebellum, but the commonest are cerebrovascular events or tumours in the posterior fossa. The causes can be summarised as follows:

1 Vascular:
- haemorrhage
- infarction
- arteriovenous malformation.

2 Tumours:
- primary brain tumours
- secondary tumours
- acoustic neuroma.

3 Infection:
- brain abscess
- human immunodeficiency virus infection.

4 Toxins:
- alcohol
- heavy metal poisoning
- solvent abuse.

Nervous system

CASE
63

5 Inherited:

- ataxia telangiectasia
- Friedreich's ataxia.

6 Others:

- multiple sclerosis
- hydrocephalus
- non-metastatic features of malignancy
- drugs (especially anticonvulsants)
- vitamin E deficiency.

Clinical features

The cerebellum is responsible for co-ordination of movement by receiving afferent nerves from proprioceptive receptors in muscles and joints and the vestibular apparatus, and sending efferent stimuli to the extrapyramidal nerve nuclei that control agonist and antagonist muscle groups to allow fine adjustment of movements. Damage to the cerebellum results in loss of this fine control and lack of co-ordination of movement (ataxia) on the same side of the body as the cerebellar damage or disease. The patient may have symptoms or signs related to the cause of the cerebellar damage (eg headache, vomiting, papilloedema associated with the presence of primary or secondary brain tumours).

Features of cerebellar dysfunction include the following:

- **Abnormal gait.** Patients often walk with a widely spaced, stamping gait, and may have a tendency to fall or veer towards the affected side.
- **Tremor and ataxia.** Because movement is not finely controlled, patients display an intention tremor and past-pointing on finger–nose testing, and are unable to perform the heel–shin test with accuracy. They cannot co-ordinate rapid alternating movements such as tapping their hand, rapid supination and pronation of the forearm or rhythmical movements of the fingers on the affected side. This condition is known as dysdiadochokinesia.
- **Speech defects.** Slurring of speech occurs due to inability to co-ordinate the muscles responsible for articulation of words and phonation. This is best demonstrated by asking the patient to repeat a phrase that contains many consonants (eg 'The British Constitution').
- **Eye signs.** Coarse horizontal nystagmus occurs with lesions of one cerebellar lobe, the fast component being towards the side of the lesion.

Nervous system

CASE
63

- **Romberg's test.** If the patient is asked to stand with their feet 4–6 inches apart, with their eyes closed, they will tend to become unsteady and to fall towards the side of the lesion, or in the case of midline cerebellar lesions to fall forwards or backwards (truncal ataxia). This test must be performed with care to ensure that the patient does not fall down and sustain injury.

Investigations

CT or MRI scans of the posterior fossa are usually necessary to determine the underlying cause. Chest X-ray may show a primary bronchogenic neoplasm, which may be associated with secondary deposits in the cerebellum, or which can cause a non-metastatic syndrome of cerebellar atrophy or dysfunction.

Treatment and management

The patient should be assessed to determine the underlying cause, and treated if at all possible. They should be referred for occupational therapy, physiotherapy and assessment for walking aids or the fitting of railings within the home to prevent falls. The patient should be advised about using visual cues as much as possible. For example, they should be told not to close their eyes while washing their face, as they would be inclined to fall over, but this will not be the case if they can visualise their surroundings.

The prognosis depends entirely on the nature of the underlying cause and the ability to correct this abnormality.

Nervous system

CASE
63

CASE 64

Testing vision and visual field defects

This clinical station is used to assess the student's ability to test visual acuity and/or determine the nature of a visual field defect. Real patients are sometimes used, but it is possible for the examiner or an actor to simulate a patient with a specific visual field defect.

Testing visual acuity

This can be done with accuracy for distance vision using a Snellen chart. The chart is placed at a position level with the patient's eyes and at a distance of six metres away. Each eye is tested in turn by covering the eye that is not being assessed. Patients should be allowed to use their normal contact lenses or spectacles for distance vision if required. The patient is asked to read the large letters from the top of the chart and to continue on to the smaller letters until they cannot identify them accurately. A record is made of the minimum size of print that is clearly seen. This is recorded in a standard fashion. For example, a visual acuity of 'left 6/12, right 6/6' indicates that distance vision in the right eye is normal, as this eye is capable of reading letters at six metres which a person with normal vision can clearly read at six metres, while the left eye has impaired vision, only being able to read letters at six metres which a person with normal vision could read clearly at 12 metres.

Near vision is assessed using standardised visual acuity charts with newsprint of various sizes written out as headlines, in large, small and very small print. Patients are asked to read these charts, and the size of print which is clearly visualised is compared with that which normal-sighted people can read.

Colour vision is assessed using Ishihara pseudoisochromatic plates. These are charts composed of a variety of coloured dots, and contained within the pattern are numbers which can be easily visualised if no colour blindness is present. By using a series of these plates with different colour combinations it is possible to determine the presence and nature of any colour blindness that may exist.

Assessment of visual fields

This is performed as a clinical test by confrontation, where the visual fields of the patient are directly compared with those of the person performing the examination. Arrange the patient and yourself so that you are seated directly opposite each other

Nervous system

CASE 64

approximately three feet apart, with your eyes looking directly at each other. To test the visual field of the patient's right eye, instruct them to cover their left eye with their left hand while you close your right eye. While the patient looks directly at your eye, move your hands in from various points in the periphery of the visual fields, equidistant from your eye and the patient's eye. Ask the patient to inform you as soon as they can see your finger moving into their visual field. This method can detect gross visual field defects.

There are nine types of visual field defect, which are associated with specific lesions of the pathway of neurones that carry impulses from the retina to the occipital cortex (see Fig 4).

Fig 4 Visual fields.

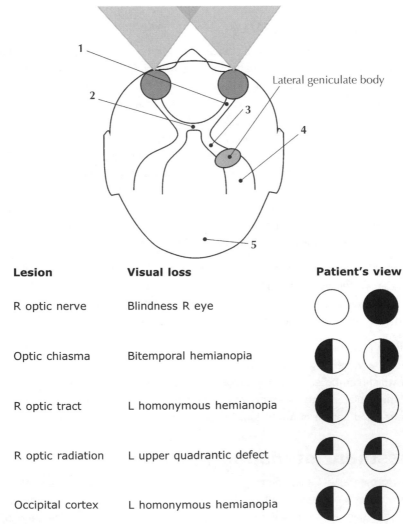

	Lesion	Visual loss	Patient's view
1	R optic nerve	Blindness R eye	
2	Optic chiasma	Bitemporal hemianopia	
3	R optic tract	L homonymous hemianopia	
4	R optic radiation	L upper quadrantic defect	
5	Occipital cortex	L homonymous hemianopia	

CASE
64

Although confrontation is an excellent clinical test for visual fields, it will only detect fairly large areas of visual field loss. A more objective and detailed assessment of visual fields can only be achieved by means of perimetry, which can detect minor areas of visual loss such as scotomas, or minor degrees of concentric narrowing of the visual field (tunnel vision).

Nervous system

CASE
64

CASE 65

The patient with impaired hearing

An important part of examination of the cranial nerves is the ability to test hearing and to differentiate between **nerve deafness**, which occurs in patients with damage to the auditory nerve (VIII), and **conductive deafness**.

In a clinical OSCE station you may be asked to show the examiner how you would assess hearing and determine the cause of any deafness. Clinical bedside or consulting-room tests of hearing are at best imprecise, and audiometry is a much more objective test of hearing. However, students should be capable of detecting impaired hearing and be able to use a tuning fork to discriminate between conductive and nerve deafness.

Assessment of hearing

This should be done in an environment that is free from other noise. Test each ear separately, and when assessing hearing stand to the side of or behind the patient so that they cannot lip-read what you are saying.

To test hearing in the left ear, occlude the patient's right ear by pressing on the skin just anterior to the external auditory meatus, and occlude the lumen of the ear canal or constantly rustle paper close to the right ear. Ask the patient to repeat the numbers that you speak. Gradually decrease the loudness of your voice to a whisper while saying the numbers until the patient is unable to repeat what you have said. Repeat the procedure in the right ear and compare the result. If hearing is impaired on one side this should be readily apparent.

If you have detected a hearing impairment, you can determine its underlying nature by using a 512 Hz tuning fork with a flat foot process and performing the Rinne and Weber tests.

Normally, sound conducted through air is heard more easily than sound transmitted via bone. This is because the ossicles of the middle ear amplify sound waves which cause the tympanic membrane to vibrate. However, if there is failure of this amplification system (conductive deafness), bone conduction is better than conduction through air.

Nervous system

CASE
65

The Weber and Rinne tests

When used in conjunction with one another, these tests can discriminate between conductive and nerve deafness as a cause of impaired hearing (see Table 15).

The Weber test

After sounding the tuning fork, place it in the centre of the patient's forehead. If their hearing is normal, the sound will be heard equally by both ears (ie in the centre of the head). If the patient only hears the sound in the left ear, this indicates that there is either nerve deafness affecting the right ear or conductive deafness on the left side. This is because in conductive deafness of the left ear all other extraneous sounds are absent, and therefore the sound transmitted via the skull bone is heard closer to the affected ear.

The Rinne test

After sounding the tuning fork, place the footplate on the mastoid process and then move it so that the forks are positioned over the external auditory meatus. In people with either normal hearing or nerve deafness, the sound is louder via air than via bone (positive Rinne test), while in those with conductive deafness the sound is louder when the tuning fork is placed on the mastoid (negative Rinne test).

Table 15 Weber and Rinne tests

	Weber test	Rinne test
Normal	Sound heard centrally	Both positive (air > bone)
Right conductive deafness	Sound heard on right side	Right negative (air < bone) Left positive (air > bone)
Right partial nerve deafness	Sound heard on left side	Left side positive Right side positive
Right complete nerve deafness	Sound heard on left side	No sound by air or bone on right side

Nervous system

CASE
65

CASE 66

Raised intracranial pressure

This is an acute medical emergency, and all doctors would be expected to recognise the clinical features of the condition. In an OSCE examination it is usually presented to the student as part of a data interpretation station where pulse, blood pressure and coma scale records are displayed.

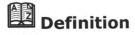 **Definition**

Raised intracranial pressure is an elevation of pressure within the cranium that causes an alteration in brain function.

? Causes

These include the following:

1 Haemorrhage:
- extradural
- subdural
- subarachnoid
- intracerebral.

2 Masses:
- primary brain tumour (benign or malignant)
- secondary brain tumour
- meningioma
- brain abscess.

3 Cerebrospinal fluid abnormalities:
- primary hydrocephalus
- secondary hydrocephalus.

Nervous system

CASE
66

4   Brain swelling:

- encephalitis
- cerebral oedema.

Clinical features

The manifestations of raised intracranial pressure depend on the rate of development of the condition, which is to some extent determined by the underlying cause. As a general rule, haemorrhage causes a rapidly rising intracranial pressure, brain masses cause a moderate rate of increase in pressure, and cerebrospinal fluid abnormalities cause a slower rise in pressure.

Papilloedema may be present on examination of the fundi (see page 201), but is not present in all patients with raised intracranial pressure. However, if papilloedema is seen in the absence of other retinal changes of arterial hypertension, you should always suspect that the patient has raised intracranial pressure.

Slowly rising intracranial pressure

In patients who develop increased pressure within the cranium over a period of many months or years, the brain has time to adjust to the increasing pressure, and symptoms may be absent. Sometimes patients have headache or complain of poor memory, and their intellectual function may deteriorate. If the condition develops in infancy or childhood, before the bones that form the cranium have fused, enlargement of the head can occur, which to some extent prevents damage to the central nervous system. Head circumference will be increased compared with children of the same age, and the IQ or academic ability will be reduced. Cranial nerve damage is uncommon.

Moderately rising intracranial pressure

In patients with brain abscess or intracranial tumours (benign or malignant) the intracranial pressure rises over a period of weeks or months. Patients complain of headache that is felt as a pressure or tension within the head and which is made worse by doing anything that further increases pressure in the head (eg stooping forward, straining at stool, sneezing or coughing). The pain may be worse in the mornings, and can be associated with vomiting (which may not be associated with nausea). Intellectual function may remain relatively normal, but there may be a change in personality or behaviour. If the mass is situated in the frontal lobe region, the patient can become disinhibited or may display antisocial behaviour. If the cause is encephalitis or brain abscess, features of fever, raised white cell count or an increase in inflammatory markers (erythrocyte sedimentation rate and C-reactive protein) will be found on investigation.

Nervous system

CASE
66

Examination of the fundi may reveal papilloedema. If the pressure is very high, cranial nerve lesions may be present (see below). If cranial nerve paralysis is present the patient may complain of double vision or blurring of vision.

Rapidly rising intracranial pressure

Classically this occurs as a result of haemorrhage, but it may be caused by acute encephalitis or acute secondary hydrocephalus. There may be a history of trauma or a fall, or the patient may be on anticoagulants or have an underlying bleeding disorder (eg chronic liver disease or thrombocytopenia).

The classic features of rising intracranial pressure are as follows:

- decreasing level of consciousness
- increasing blood pressure
- decreasing pulse rate
- development of cranial nerve signs (the third cranial nerve is most often affected).

As the pressure rises the patient starts to complain of headache, which is felt as a severe pain or bursting pressure within the head. They start to become drowsy and then lapse into unconsciousness, which gets progressively deeper as reflected by a decreasing score on the Glasgow Coma Scale (see page 154).

Routine observations show that the pulse rate progressively falls and the blood pressure rises in response to the increasing pressure in the brain. As the pressure increases further, cranial nerves that have a long intracranial course may become damaged. This is particularly likely to occur in the case of the third cranial nerve, which can become compressed as it hooks over the tentorium cerebelli. The effect is best illustrated by considering the classic history and clinical features of an extradural haematoma.

Extradural haematoma

This usually occurs as a result of trauma to the temporal region of the skull (eg a fall that involves hitting the side of the head on the ground). The initial trauma may cause loss of consciousness which is regained. If there is haemorrhage from the middle meningeal artery into the subdural space, the intracranial pressure rises rapidly, causing the patient to become drowsy and then lapse into unconsciousness. The period during which the patient was conscious is known as the lucid interval. As the size of the haematoma increases, the pressure on the brain rises, the pulse rate falls and the blood pressure starts to rise progressively. The pressure on the same

CASE
66

Nervous system

side of the brain as the haematoma causes irritation of the third cranial nerve as it becomes pressed against the tentorium on that side, and this results in constriction of the pupil. As the pressure rises further, the nerve becomes paralysed and the pupil dilates. As the pressure rises even further, the cranial nerve on the opposite side becomes compressed and constriction of the pupil on the opposite side to the subdural haematoma occurs. A further rise in pressure causes paralysis of this nerve and fixed dilated pupils are then present bilaterally. If the pressure is not immediately relieved by surgical evacuation of the haematoma, it causes **coning** of the brain with respiratory centre damage and eventual respiratory arrest and death.

A respiratory sign of critically high intracranial pressure is the Cheyne-Stokes pattern of respiration. When present, this is associated with a very poor prognosis.

Investigations

Every patient with suspected raised intracranial pressure should have an emergency CT or MRI scan of the brain to identify the underlying cause so that definitive therapy can be planned. Additional investigations such as a full blood picture, white cell count, differential white cell count, blood cultures, erythrocyte sedimentation rate, C-reactive protein, coagulation screen and liver function tests are performed to try to identify what other conditions might be associated with or causing the condition.

If raised intracranial pressure is suspected, **the patient must not have lumbar puncture performed**, as this can result in sudden death due to coning of the brain. It is wise to arrange for CT or MRI scans of all patients before lumbar puncture is performed, and only to proceed when raised Intracranial pressure has been conclusively ruled out.

Treatment

Emergency surgical management

If intracranial pressure is rising rapidly it must be reduced. In cases of haemorrhage this usually requires surgical drainage or evacuation of the haematoma. If the cause is sudden accumulation of cerebrospinal fluid under pressure, a shunt can be inserted to drain the fluid from one of the ventricles of the brain into the peritoneal cavity.

Medical treatments to reduce raised intracranial pressure

- If the underlying cause is infection (eg encephalitis, meningitis or abscess), antiviral or antibacterial drug therapy should be administered intravenously at a high dose.

Nervous system

CASE
66

- Provided that infection has been ruled out, intracranial pressure can be reduced to some degree by the use of steroid therapy (dexamethasone, 10 mg initially followed by 4 mg to 8 mg orally or by intravenous injection every six hours for 48–72 hours.

- Mannitol infusion increases the osmotic pressure of the blood and causes the movement of fluid from brain cells into the bloodstream, thus reducing the pressure within the head. The dose is 200 mg per kg body weight, given as a 20% mannitol solution infused over 24 hours.

Nervous system

CASE
66

The eye

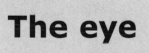

CASE 67

Hypertensive retinopathy and papilloedema

Examination of the fundus using an ophthalmoscope is a common clinical station. Because large numbers of students are usually being assessed in an OSCE examination, these clinical stations commonly involve mannequin heads designed specifically for the purpose. Only the following pathological conditions are used:

- hypertensive retinopathy
- papilloedema
- diabetic retinopathy
- optic atrophy.

For all of these the student must show that they are competent in the use of the ophthalmoscope, capable of visualising both of the patient's eyes without causing discomfort, and able to quickly detect any abnormality that is present.

It will always impress the examiner if you have your own ophthalmoscope with you, but make sure that you know how to use it properly. Talk to the mannequin as if you were talking to a real patient and, before you examine the fundus, briefly explain to the 'patient' what you are going to do. Let the examiner see that you inspect all of the fundus, including the peripheral regions of the retina. Do not take too long to examine each eye, and if you then arrive at your diagnosis, having ensured that you have looked for all of the possible changes, tell the examiner what it is and list the features. It is always desirable to show that when you perform a comprehensive examination you are capable of reaching a diagnosis quickly.

The eye

CASE 67

Hypertensive retinopathy

This is a common clinical examination station, and it represents an important aspect of the assessment of any patient with raised blood pressure.

Four grades or degrees of hypertensive retinopathy occur in patients with long-standing hypertension. The degree of retinopathy correlates with the severity and duration of the hypertension (see Fig 5).

Fig 5 Hypertensive retinopathy.

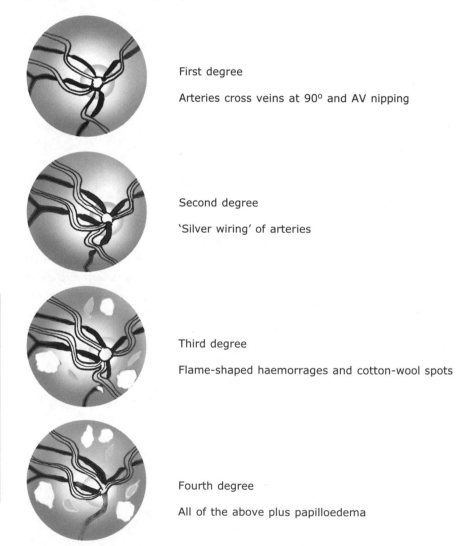

First degree

Arteries cross veins at 90° and AV nipping

Second degree

'Silver wiring' of arteries

Third degree

Flame-shaped haemorrages and cotton-wool spots

Fourth degree

All of the above plus papilloedema

The eye

CASE
67

First degree

Normally the retinal arteries and veins run side by side and the arteries cross the veins at an acute angle. The raised arterial pressure results in thickening of the muscular wall of the arteries, and the earliest visible changes consist of the arteries crossing the veins at 90° and compressing the underlying vein, giving the latter the appearance of being 'nipped' by the artery.

Second degree

As the arterial wall thickens further, the arteries develop an appearance similar to that of an insulated electrical wire which has been stripped. The central core of red blood appears like the wire, and the thickened white arterial wall resembles the layer of insulation around the wire. This appearance is termed 'silver wiring' or 'copper wiring'.

Third degree

At higher pressures, small haemorrhages can occur in the superficial layers of the retina. These take on the shape of candle or matchstick flames, and are termed 'flame-shaped haemorrhages'. Other areas of the retina become ischaemic due to the very high pressure, causing some small arterioles to become occluded. These ischaemic areas are termed 'cotton-wool spots' because of their white fluffy appearance. In some textbooks you may see them referred to as 'soft exudates', but this is a misnomer as they are areas of ischaemia and not due to exudation.

Fourth degree

The development of papilloedema superimposed on the other features is an extremely serious and sinister clinical feature, and it indicates very severe hypertension that requires urgent treatment. Papilloedema is diagnosed by loss of the physiological cup in the optic nerve head, an indistinct edge to the optic nerve, loss of normal venous pulsation of the veins approaching the optic nerve, and bulging of the optic nerve head.

Papilloedema

The presence of papilloedema without any of the other features of hypertensive retinopathy is an extremely important clinical sign, as it indicates raised intracranial pressure.

In papilloedema the optic nerve head is pink and swollen and has blurred margins. Small haemorrhages may be seen at the margins of the optic disc.

The eye

**CASE
67**

Causes of papilloedema include the following:

- intracranial space-occupying lesion
- obstructive hydrocephalus
- cerebral venous thrombosis.

The eye

CASE
67

CASE 68

Diabetic retinopathy

This extremely common condition is frequently used in OSCE examinations, and it is important that young doctors can identify the early signs of retinal damage in a patient, as well as being able to recognise features that indicate impending visual impairment.

Clinical features

Microaneurysms

These are small aneurysms which occur on the retinal arteries.

Dot and blot haemorrhages

Because the bleeds occur in the deeper layers of the retina, they form discrete well-demarcated dots and blots of various sizes scattered in various regions of the retina.

Hard exudates

These are yellowish-white exudates which, unlike the cotton-wool spots of hypertensive retinopathy, form well-demarcated areas due to the fact that they are held in the deeper retinal layers.

Neovascularisation

This occurs in areas of retinal ischaemia due to the liberation of growth factors that stimulate angiogenesis. When this is present it is termed **proliferative retinopathy**. The new vessels are fragile because they lack adequate connective tissue support and can bleed easily, causing vitreous haemorrhage, and the formation of fibrous bands, which can lead to retinal detachment.

Neovascularisation is often treated with laser photocoagulation, and it is important to be able to recognise these characteristic, well-circumscribed areas of 'laser burns', which may be seen in real diabetic patients encountered in the examination.

The eye

CASE 68

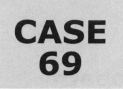

CASE 69

Optic atrophy

Definition

In optic atrophy the optic disc is pale or white with a very discrete margin. The patient's visual acuity is invariably reduced.

? Causes

A number of medical conditions can lead to optic atrophy, but the commonest is demyelinating disease, especially multiple sclerosis. In the early stages one may see only pallor of the temporal margin of the discs, and this is a very useful clinical sign which should suggest the possibility of multiple sclerosis in any patient presenting with transient neurological symptoms.

Medical causes of optic atrophy include the following:

- demyelinating disease (eg multiple sclerosis)
- retrobulbar neuritis
- optic nerve compression (pituitary tumours)
- central retinal artery occlusion (diabetes, arteriosclerosis or vasculitis)
- secondary to papilloedema
- vitamin B_{12} deficiency
- toxins (tobacco, methyl alcohol, heavy metals).

Clinical features

The patient may have other clinical features associated with the underlying cause. All cases have some impairment of visual acuity, often with a visual field defect. Complete optic atrophy results in blindness in the affected eye with loss of the direct light reflex in that eye and loss of the consensual reflex in the other eye. In less severe forms, the visual field defect depends on the extent of the optic nerve damage and to some extent on the underlying cause. For example, following retrobulbar neuritis there may be a residual central scotoma while multiple sclerosis can cause arcuate scotomas ranging in size.

The eye

CASE 69

Investigations

These are directed at trying to determine the underlying cause and include CT or MRI scans of the brain to identify demyelination, pituitary tumours or other space-occupying lesions causing raised intracranial pressure.

Detailed investigation of the visual acuity and visual fields using perimetry will determine the extent of the visual impairment and may give a clue as to the possible underlying cause.

Treatment

Once optic nerve damage has occurred, recovery is unlikely and therefore treatment of the underlying medical condition will only prevent any further deterioration in vision.

The eye

CASE
69

Endocrinology/metabolic medicine

CASE 70

Diabetes mellitus

This common condition, which affects 1% of the population, may be encountered at a history-taking station with a patient complaining of thirst or polyuria, or at a data interpretation station where blood sugar results or glucose tolerance tests are to be interpreted. Students are expected to have a good working knowledge of how the condition should be diagnosed and managed, and of the various complications.

Definition and classification

Diabetes mellitus is a chronic condition characterised by hyperglycaemia due to a deficiency of insulin production by the pancreas, or a state of insulin resistance.

There are two forms of diabetes mellitus:

1 **Type 1 (insulin-dependent) diabetes** is due to an absolute deficiency of insulin production by the beta islet cells of the pancreas. This condition can occur at any age, but usually presents under the age of 40 years, and is more common in men than in women.

2 **Type 2 (non-insulin-dependent) diabetes** (formerly known as maturity-onset diabetes) usually presents over the age of 40 years, and is more common in women than in men. It can be controlled to some degree by dietary measures and the use of oral hypoglycaemic drugs, but patients may need to be treated with insulin as the disorder can progressively worsen.

Secondary diabetes

Any condition that causes damage to the pancreas, thereby impairing insulin production, or any condition that increases the blood sugar level can lead to hyperglycaemia. The causes of secondary diabetes include the following:

- chronic pancreatitis
- pancreatic carcinoma
- haemochromatosis

CASE 70

- acromegaly
- Cushing's syndrome
- phaeochromocytoma
- thyrotoxicosis
- pregnancy
- cirrhosis of the liver
- hepatitis
- drugs (eg thiazide diuretics, steroids)
- pancreatectomy.

Clinical features

High levels of glucose in the blood cause an osmotic diuresis with the passage of large quantities of urine (polyuria). As a result of this, and also because the high level of glucose makes the blood hyperosmolar, the patient feels very thirsty and starts drinking large quantities of fluids (polydipsia). Their thirst is pathological, and is commonly so severe that they waken at night feeling thirsty, and they often report taking drinks (eg large bottles of water) to bed so that they can drink through the night. In type 1 diabetes, the patient becomes thin as a result of fluid loss and the breakdown of fat as a source of energy. The metabolism of fat results in the production of ketones in the bloodstream. If the rate of ketone production exceeds the rate of clearance, the excess is exhaled, giving a characteristic acetone fetor.

In type 2 diabetes, because the patient has normal or even high levels of circulating insulin they do not show the same degree of weight loss. Indeed they often show a considerable weight gain and become markedly obese. They do not tend to break down fat to the same extent, and are less likely to have the fetor associated with insulin-dependent diabetes.

Many of the clinical features of diabetes are due to the complications that can arise from hyperglycaemia. The latter is associated with pathological changes in blood vessels, and the complications of diabetes are mainly a result of **macrovascular complications**. The resulting arteriosclerosis can lead to hypertension, ischaemic heart disease, peripheral vascular disease and cerebral ischaemia or cerebrovascular events.

Microvascular complications occur as a consequence of damage to the small blood vessels of the kidney, retina and nerves, resulting in renal disease (eg protein loss and diabetic glomerulosclerosis), retinopathy (with the development of microaneurysms, haemorrhages and exudates) and damage to peripheral nerves (causing motor, sensory or autonomic neuropathy).

CASE
70

The combination of peripheral vascular insufficiency and loss of sensation in peripheral tissues can lead to skin changes and impaired healing, so that the patient may develop foot and leg ulcers which fail to heal, can become quite extensive and may lead to peripheral gangrene.

Investigations

The diagnosis of diabetes mellitus is usually straightforward. An elevated random blood sugar level of > 11 mmol/litre on two or more occasions, or a fasting blood sugar level of > 7 mmol/litre in two or more samples, is diagnostic.

A glucose tolerance test is used in borderline cases. In this test, an adult is given 75 g of glucose dissolved in 300 ml of water, after a fasting blood sample (for glucose) has been taken. A further blood sample is taken two hours after the glucose drink. Diabetes is diagnosed on the basis of a fasting level of > 7 mmol/litre or a level of > 11 mmol/litre in the blood sample taken two hours after the glucose load.

Urine testing, although it can be suggestive of diabetes, is not highly specific as some glucose may appear in the urine in normal individuals after a large glucose load in a meal or drink. Some people have a low renal threshold for glucose excretion and may have mild glycosuria but normal blood sugar levels.

Two of the major complications of diabetes mellitus, particularly insulin-dependent diabetes, are hyperglycaemia with ketoacidosis and hypoglycaemia. Both of these conditions are acute medical emergencies, and students are expected to know how they are diagnosed and managed.

Treatment

For both type 1 and type 2 diabetes, patients are started on a low-fat, high-fibre, low-refined-carbohydrate diet. Strict calorie control is used to encourage weight reduction in type 2 patients. In some patients with type 2 diabetes this is sufficient to bring the blood sugar level to within or close to the normal range, and this is all that is required. If the blood sugar level remains unacceptably high, three main groups of hypoglycaemic drugs can be used:

1 **Sulphonylureas.** These stimulate the production of insulin by the beta islet cells of the pancreas, and are used to reduce the blood sugar level.

2 **Biguanides.** These increase peripheral uptake of sugar into the cells and have an insulin-like action, but are not dependent on the insulin receptor for uptake of glucose.

3 **Glitazones.** This group of drugs can be used to reduce insulin resistance.

CASE
70

For patients with type 1 diabetes mellitus, the treatment is insulin replacement therapy using short-acting, long-acting or a combination of short- and long-acting insulin drugs to achieve good blood sugar control over a 24-hour period. Blood sugar control can be assessed using a glycosylated haemoglobin (Hb A_{1C}) test, which gives a measure of glycaemic control over a period of 6–8 weeks. Patients are also encouraged to monitor their capillary blood sugar levels and make appropriate adjustments to their insulin dosage.

A type 1 diabetic patient's blood sugar level is dependent on three main factors, and if these are in balance, variations in blood sugar concentration can be kept to an acceptable level:

1 **Dietary intake of carbohydrate.** Patients should eat regular meals and have a carbohydrate intake that is relatively constant each day.

2 **Level of physical activity.** If patients expend too much energy (eg as a result of playing sport), they will use up many calories and their blood sugar level will fall. Conversely, if they rest and expend little or no energy, their blood sugar level will rise.

3 **Dose of insulin.** If dietary intake and level of physical activity remain constant, the dose of insulin required will remain constant. However, patients can adjust the insulin dose to allow for variations in dietary intake and/or physical activity and monitor their glycaemic control by capillary blood sugar testing.

There is strong evidence that strict control of blood sugar levels results in a lower risk of complications in diabetes mellitus, and therefore patients should be strongly encouraged to keep their blood sugar level within acceptable limits and to attend a diabetic clinic regularly so that any complications which may arise can be detected and treated promptly.

CASE
70

CASE 71

Diabetes insipidus

This is a rare condition, but it must be considered as a differential diagnosis at a history-taking station with a patient complaining of polyuria and polydipsia. It may also be encountered at a data interpretation station where blood and urine biochemical results or specific gravity measurements are presented to the student.

Definition and classification

Diabetes insipidus is a disorder associated with the excretion of excessive quantities of urine of low specific gravity, and with thirst.

There are two types of diabetes insipidus:

1 It may be due to decreased production of antidiuretic hormone (ADH) as a result of damage to the posterior pituitary gland by trauma, pituitary or suprapituitary tumours, or as a result of skull fracture or inflammation of the meninges at the base of the brain.

2 Nephrogenic diabetes insipidus is a rare genetic disease in which blood levels of antidiuretic hormone are normal, but the distal renal tubules and collecting ducts are unresponsive to the hormone.

Clinical features

Patients with diabetes insipidus describe polyuria and polydipsia, and pass between 5 and 20 litres of urine daily. The resulting dehydration means that they are constantly thirsty and drink large volumes of fluid each day. The specific gravity of the urine remains low, as they are unable to concentrate it. If they fail to maintain their fluid intake they become severely dehydrated.

🔍 Investigations

The patient will pass large volumes of urine even when they are fluid-restricted, and the specific gravity of their urine remains within the range 0.002–0.004, even on a fluid restriction regime. The failure to concentrate the urine is diagnostic, but the test must be performed carefully, as patients can become severely dehydrated during the course of a prolonged fluid deprivation test.

Differential diagnosis

The more common causes of polyuria and polydipsia are diabetes mellitus or hypercalcaemia.

💊 Treatment

ADH deficiency is treated by replacement therapy using vasopressin. This is a synthetic agent with a similar action to antidiuretic hormone. It can be given either as a slow-release intramuscular or subcutaneous injection, or is more commonly administered as a nasal spray. Nephrogenic diabetes insipidus does not respond to vasopressin and requires careful fluid and electrolyte balance.

CASE
71

CASE 72

Hypercalcaemia

This condition must be considered at a history-taking station where the patient complains of polyuria and polydipsia. It may also be encountered at a data interpretation station where a biochemical profile is displayed.

📖 Definition

Hypercalcaemia is characterised by an elevated level of calcium in the blood.

❓ Causes

The condition has a number of causes, but the commonest is secondary malignancy affecting the bones. Primary hyperparathyroidism is the second commonest cause.

The main causes of hypercalcaemia can be summarised as follows:

- secondary malignancy in bone
- primary hyperparathyroidism
- sarcoidosis
- ectopic parathormone production (small-cell cancer)
- production of osteoclast-activating factor from tumours (especially myeloma)
- vitamin D intoxication
- milk-alkali syndrome
- bone resorption phase of Paget's disease
- prolonged immobility
- tertiary hyperparathyroidism
- familial hypocalciuric hypercalcaemia.

Endocrinology

📝 Clinical features

As a result of high levels of calcium in the blood, deposits of calcium salts can occur in the skin, subcutaneous tissues and internal organs. Intracellular calcium levels rise and cell function is impaired. This is seen in particular in muscle cells, the cells of the nervous system and of the gastrointestinal tract, cardiac cells and the renal tubules.

Musculoskeletal symptoms

Muscle relaxation is inhibited and the patient experiences muscle stiffness and lethargy. Bone pain and spontaneous or pathological fractures occur if the underlying cause is malignancy or hyperparathyroidism.

Neurological symptoms

Brain function is altered as a result of the high level of calcium. The patient may be confused, have a personality change or become psychotic. In severe cases, the level of consciousness may be impaired or coma may develop.

Gastrointestinal symptoms

Constipation and/or crampy abdominal pains are common. Anorexia, nausea and vomiting may also occur.

Renal symptoms

The deposition of calcium salts in renal tissues (nephrocalcinosis) and the high urinary calcium levels can result in renal calculus formation, and the patient may develop renal colic. Because of the impaired renal tubular function, polyuria and polydipsia occur. In severe or prolonged hypercalcaemia, acute or chronic renal failure may develop.

Cardiac features

With mild to moderate elevation of serum calcium levels, the ECG may show a shortened QT interval. In severe cases, when the serum calcium concentration exceeds 4 mmol/litre) sudden cardiac arrest may occur.

Collectively, the features of hypercalcaemia can be remembered by the phrase 'Too much calcium causes pains in the bones, abdominal groans, psychiatric moans and renal stones'.

CASE
72

Endocrinology

Investigations

The condition is diagnosed on the basis of a corrected serum calcium level above the upper limit of normal (> 2.6 mmol/litre) after a correction has been made for the serum albumin level. Further investigations are then directed at finding the underlying cause, and include the following:

1 chest X-ray and skeletal survey – to look for lung tumour or evidence of secondary bony deposits

2 radioisotope bone scan – to look for increased isotope uptake ('hot spots') which occurs with malignant deposits

3 serum parathormone assay – to investigate the possibility of primary or tertiary hyperparathyroidism

4 angiotension-converting-enzyme (ACE) assay – which is elevated in sarcoidosis

5 serum immunoglobulins and urinary electrophoresis – to identify a monoclonal antibody or urinary Bence Jones proteins which would suggest multiple myeloma

6 plain X-ray of the abdomen – which may reveal calcification of the kidneys

7 CT scan of the abdomen – to look for a solid tumour of the kidney or pancreas, or secondary liver deposits

8 prostate-specific antigen (PSA) – to detect a prostatic tumour.

Treatment

For mild cases, the use of intravenous fluids (3–5 litres/24 hours) to replace fluid loss furosemide and 20 mg 6–8 times daily to encourage urinary calcium excretion are often helpful. Oral bisphosphonates can be used to encourage calcium uptake into the bones. For hypercalcaemia of malignancy, sarcoidosis or vitamin D toxicity, the use of corticosteroids (prednisolone 60 mg daily) is often effective.

Patients with hyperparathyroidism often do not respond to steroid therapy, and surgical resection of the parathyroid adenoma is usually required.

In severe cases (serum calcium concentration > 3.5 mmol/litre), urgent treatment is required to reduce the risk of cardiac arrest. Large volumes of 0.9% saline (5–6 litres/24 hours) together with furosemide 40–60 mg administered intravenously every 2–4 hours may be required. However, electrolyte balance must be carefully monitored. Magnesium chloride (20 mmol infused over 12 hours) or the use of bisphosphonate infusion may be necessary for severe cases.

CASE
72

Endocrinology

If these measures are not effective, peritoneal dialysis or haemodialysis may be required. If the underlying cause is determined and amenable to correction, this should be achieved. This is usually possible for patients with primary hyperparathyroidism, milk-alkali syndrome, sarcoidosis, vitamin D overdose or chronic immobilisation.

Hypercalcaemia in patients with malignancy is less easily controlled, and naturally these patients have a much worse prognosis.

CASE
72

Endocrinology

CASE 73

Hyperthyroidism

This condition is usually encountered at a clinical examination station where the student is shown a photograph of a patient with the classic eye changes of hyperthyroidism.

📖 Definition

Hyperthyroidism is a condition characterised by over-production of thyroxine by the thyroid gland.

📝 Clinical features

Hyperthyroidism is more common in women than in men. Patients show a variety of clinical features which are due to the action of thyroxine increasing the metabolic rate. The classic features are weight loss with an excellent appetite, a fine tremor of the outstretched hands, sweating, palpitations, heat intolerance, episodes of diarrhoea, and enlargement of the thyroid gland.

There are a number of characteristic signs which can be seen on inspection of the eyes, including exophthalmos (also known as exophthalmicproptosis), lid lag, lid retraction and, in severe cases, ophthalmoplegia.

- **Lid lag.** Normally when the eye moves from an upward to a downward gaze, the upper lid closely follows the downward movement. In thyrotoxicosis there is a delay in the upper lid movement.

- **Lid retraction.** Normally when the upper eyelid is in its resting position, no sclera is visible above the iris. In hyperthyroid patients the upper lid is retracted and the sclera is clearly seen.

Excess circulating thyroxine levels can cause atrial fibrillation, and an irregularly irregular pulse may be present. As a result of weight loss, women with hyperthyroidism may develop oligomenorrhoea or amenorrhoea.

🔍 Investigations

The serum thyroxine level will be elevated above the normal range, and the level of thyroid-stimulating hormone (TSH) will be below the normal range.

CASE 73

Treatment

Before specific therapy is effective, patients who have palpitations may require β-blocker therapy to reduce the symptoms associated with tachycardia.

Three forms of antithyroid therapy can be used to treat hyperthyroidism.

Drug therapy

Antithyroid drugs are used to suppress the production of thyroxine in the gland. Most of them are thiourea derivatives that block the incorporation of iodine into the organic precursors of the thyroid hormones T3 (tri-iodothyronine) and T4 (thyroxine).

1 **Carbimazole suppression.** In most cases, symptoms improve within 7–10 days of treatment with this drug, but it can take up to eight weeks before the patient's thyroxine level is reduced to normal. The dose can be gradually adjusted to maintain an acceptable level of thyroxine which prevents symptoms.

2 **Block and replacement therapy.** It can sometimes be difficult to adjust the level of thyroxine accurately using carbimazole alone. Therefore, in most patients, the endogenous thyroxine production can be blocked completely using a high dose of carbimazole, followed by thyroxine replacement therapy to achieve a thyroxine level that is within the normal range.

Surgery

Partial or total thyroidectomy can be performed, and is particularly indicated for patients with a large goitre. Pre-operative potassium iodide is used to reduce the level of serum thyroxine and also to decrease the vascularity of the gland prior to surgical intervention. After treatment, thyroid hormone replacement therapy may be required, and there is also a risk that damage to the blood supply to the parathyroid glands may lead to transient or permanent hypoparathyroidism.

Radioactive iodine

Iodine is avidly taken up by thyroid tissue. Therefore the radioactive isotope I^{131} can be used to selectively ablate thyroid cells. In 50% of patients who are treated in this way hypothyroidism will develop, although this can be delayed for many months or years.

CASE
73

CASE 74

Hypothyroidism

This metabolic disorder has a variety of clinical symptoms and signs, and may be encountered at history-taking or clinical examination stations.

Definition

Hypothyroidism is a deficiency of thyroid hormone that results in a reduction in metabolic rate and a slowing of all bodily functions and activity.

? Causes

In most patients the underlying cause is an autoimmune reaction which causes inflammation and destruction of thyroid hormone-producing cells or the production of autoantibodies that are responsible for blocking thyroid-stimulating hormone (TSH) receptors and inhibiting thyroxine production. The main causes are:

- autoimmune anti-TSH-receptor antibodies
- autoimmune antithyroid antibodies
- Hashimoto's thyroiditis
- post-thyroidectomy or after radioactive iodine
- iodine deficiency
- carcinoma of thyroid.

Clinical features

The main symptoms are as follows:

- weight gain
- cold intolerance
- menorrhagia
- dry, brittle, sparse, coarse hair
- constipation
- lack of energy.

CASE
74

On physical examination, the classic features are as follows:

- coarse features with or without goitre
- loss of the outer third of the eyebrow
- bradycardia
- reduced intellectual agility
- perifollicular keratosis
- 'hung-up' reflexes (ie slow relaxation phase).

Investigations

A reduced serum thyroxine level with an elevated TSH level is diagnostic of primary hypothyroidism.

Patients often have a raised serum cholesterol level, and the creatine kinase concentration may be extremely high.

Antithyroid antibodies may be detected in those patients in whom autoimmune thyroid antibodies are responsible for the thyroid cell destruction.

Treatment

Thyroxine replacement therapy should be given. Initially L-thyroxine 50 micrograms daily is given. The dose is slowly increased over a period of 4–6 weeks to a maintenance dose which is sufficient to keep the serum thyroxine concentration at the upper level of normal and the TSH level within the normal range (100–150 micrograms daily is usually sufficient for the majority of patients).

CASE
74

CASE 75

Addison's disease (hypoadrenalism)

This is an uncommon condition, but because it is a cause of fainting or syncopal attacks it may be encountered at a history-taking station. Several classic skin changes occur in association with this condition, and therefore it may also be encountered at a station showing a photograph of a patient with increased pigmentation over the extensor surfaces of the limbs.

Definition

Addison's disease is defined as primary adrenocortical insufficiency with reduced production of corticosteroids and mineralocorticoids.

Causes

This condition is usually due to a primary autoimmune disease in which antibodies against the cells of the adrenal cortex result in atrophy and therefore failure of production of the adrenal corticosteroids. The second commonest cause is tuberculous infection. The condition may also be due to metastatic deposits of cancer, the commonest site of the primary tumour being the lung. Occasionally both adrenal glands are removed because of secondary tumour deposits, and naturally this results in complete adrenal insufficiency.

Clinical features

The onset of this condition is usually insidious, and most often presents in those aged 30–50 years, with symptoms of tiredness, weakness and weight loss. The patient then develops episodes of fainting due to hypotension. The systolic blood pressure is usually less than 100 mmHg. Skin creases become pigmented, and there is hyperpigmentation over extensor surfaces, such as the skin over the elbows and the knees. There is also increased pigmentation of the mucous membrane of the mouth beside the second upper premolar.

Addisonian crisis is a condition in which failure of corticosteroid production in response to infection, trauma (including surgery) or any intercurrent illness causes profound symptoms of nausea and vomiting, muscle weakness and abdominal pain, and is associated with low blood pressure and low serum sodium levels.

Investigations

Because of the deficiency or absence of mineralocorticoids, resorption of sodium in the kidney is suppressed and therefore the serum sodium concentration is markedly reduced. Failure to reabsorb sodium results in excessive water loss, and the blood urea and serum creatinine levels may be elevated. Measurement of the serum cortisol concentration will reveal a marked deficiency, and there is loss of the usual diurnal variation.

The best diagnostic test is the Synacthen^R stimulation test. A blood sample is taken for measurement of the serum cortisol level, and the patient is then injected with 1 mg of Synacthen^R (synthetic adrenocorticotropic hormone or ACTH). A further blood sample is taken 30 minutes after the injection. In normal individuals, the synthetic ACTH stimulation will cause a doubling of the serum cortisol level in the 30-minute sample, whereas failure to produce an increase in the cortisol concentration indicates adrenal insufficiency.

Treatment

Replacement therapy using hydrocortisone 25–50 mg daily given in divided doses (eg 12.5 mg twice daily) replaces the deficiency of endogenous cortisol. If the patient's serum sodium level fails to increase, the mineralocorticoid fludrocortisone should be given at a dose of 0.1–0.3 mg each day.

The patient should be warned that if they are to undergo any surgical procedure or during the course of any physical illness, particularly infection, they should increase their dose of hydrocortisone.

Treatment of addisonian crisis

If the patient presents with acute addisonian crisis, large volumes of intravenous 0.9% saline together with dextrose infusion should be given. Hydrocortisone 100 mg should be given intravenously every eight hours, and fluid and electrolyte balance must be carefully monitored. Any underlying cause should be treated promptly.

CASE
75

CASE 76

Cushing's syndrome

This condition may be encountered at a clinical examination station with a real patient or a clinical photograph, as Cushing's syndrome can often be diagnosed on general inspection.

Definition

This is a metabolic disorder that results from chronic excess of glucocorticoids.

Causes

A number of conditions can result in increased levels of steroids in the circulation. The commonest cause is iatrogenic, due to the prescribing of steroid hormones such as prednisone or prednisolone. A less common cause is Cushing's disease, which is due to a pituitary adenoma.

The main causes of Cushing's syndrome can be summarised as follows:

- iatrogenic causes (steroid drug treatment)
- Cushing's disease (adenoma of the pituitary)
- adrenal adenoma
- adrenal carcinoma
- ectopic adrenocorticotropic hormone (ACTH) production.

Clinical features

The features of the disease are due to the excessive action of corticosteroids which increase protein breakdown, reduce the inflammatory response in the body, promote sodium retention and potassium excretion, increase gluconeogenesis and alter calcium metabolism.

The patient develops central obesity with wasting of both muscle and fat tissue on the limbs. They have impaired glucose tolerance, and 20% of patients develop symptoms and signs of diabetes. Because of the sodium retention, high blood pressure can occur, muscle wasting develops and the patient may describe proximal

Endocrinology

muscle weakness. They characteristically develop a rounded face (moon face), and there is increased accumulation of brown fat at the nape of the neck (buffalo hump), and thin skin, with the patient bruising easily and prone to infection.

The skeletal bones become osteoporotic, and the patient is at increased risk of fractures.

Investigations

The diagnosis is usually suspected on the basis of the general appearance of the patient, and often there will be a history of steroid therapy, either at high dosage or over a prolonged period of time. In patients who develop features of Cushing's syndrome without a history of drug treatment with steroids, the possibility of an underlying pituitary or adrenal cause should be investigated. The urine may show increased levels of urinary free cortisol, and the serum cortisol concentration is elevated in this condition. The adrenal and pituitary causes can be determined using a combination of the high-dose and low-dose dexamethasone suppression tests, together with measurement of ACTH and cortisol levels.

Treatment

If the disease is due to steroid drug treatment, an effort should be made to reduce the dose of steroids if possible. This can sometimes be achieved by using a steroid-sparing drug, such as azathioprine. Pituitary adenomas are treated by surgery or pituitary irradiation. Adrenal tumours require adrenalectomy with post-operative steroid replacement therapy. If Cushing's syndrome is a result of ectopic ACTH production, such as occurs in some forms of lung cancer, removal of the primary lung tumour is corrective.

CASE
76

Endocrinology

CASE 77

Conn's syndrome

This is an extremely rare cause of high blood pressure, but because it has a characteristic biochemical profile it may be encountered at a data interpretation station.

Definition

Conn's syndrome is defined as primary hyperaldosteronism as a result of over-production of aldosterone by the adrenal cortex, usually due to the presence of an adrenal adenoma or, less often, to adrenal hyperplasia.

Clinical features

This condition can occur at any age, but is more common in adulthood, and the female:male ratio is 2:1. It usually presents as hypertension (1% of all patients with hypertension have a raised blood pressure due to Conn's syndrome).

Because of the increased circulating levels of aldosterone, sodium and water retention occurs in the kidneys, and this is responsible for the increased blood pressure (due to an increase in blood volume). For each sodium ion that is resorbed, one ion of either potassium or hydrogen is excreted in the urine. Therefore patients with this condition characteristically have a low serum potassium concentration, and because of the excretion of hydrogen ions they become alkalotic. This can result in muscle spasm similar to tetany.

Because of the low serum potassium concentration, ventricular arrhythmias can occur, the ECG may show flattening of the T waves, and the patient may develop hypokalaemic nephropathy. As a result of the hypertension, all of the complications of raised blood pressure, including hypertensive cardiac failure, cerebrovascular accident and renal impairment, can develop.

CASE 77

Endocrinology

Investigations

Any patient with raised blood pressure who is found to have a low serum potassium level and a high pH or other features of alkalosis should be further investigated for possible Conn's syndrome. High circulating levels of aldosterone can be detected, and renal or adrenal vein sampling can be performed to show whether the increased production of aldosterone is from one or both adrenal glands.

Treatment

If the cause is adrenal adenoma, surgical resection is curative. If the cause is adrenal hyperplasia, removal of one adrenal gland will reduce the degree of hypertension. Blood pressure that is not well controlled should be treated with antihypertensive drugs and diuretics. Spironolactone, which is an aldosterone antagonist, is particularly useful.

CASE
77

Musculoskeletal disorders

CASE 78

Rheumatoid arthritis

This is an extremely common clinical station, as there are plenty of patients available who exhibit changes due to chronic rheumatoid arthritis in the hands.

Definition

Rheumatoid arthritis is a systemic disease of unknown cause which is mainly manifested by chronic inflammation of synovial membranes that leads to a deforming arthropathy. It affects 1–3% of the population, and is twice as common in women as in men. The peak age at onset is 20–40 years.

Clinical features

This condition usually has an insidious onset. Patients initially describe stiffness of the joints, mainly affecting the small joints of the hands but also affecting the toes and larger joints, such as the wrists, elbows and knees. The patient then goes on to develop a symmetrical polyarthritis with pain and stiffness, which is worse in the morning. They may also have constitutional symptoms, such as fatigue, reduced appetite and general malaise. On clinical examination during the acute inflammatory phase, the joints are swollen, hot to the touch, tender, and have limitation of movement. As the disease progresses there is destruction of the synovial structures, the ligaments and the tendons around the joint, and a deforming arthritis results, with atrophy of the muscles surrounding the inflamed joints. Extra-articular features include skin ulcers, digital ischaemia, pleural effusions, pulmonary fibrosis and splenomegaly. Patients often develop rheumatoid nodules, which are most commonly found on the extensor aspects of the elbow joints over the olecranon process, but may also be found around the wrist joint or on the dorsum of the hand. The presence of rheumatoid nodules indicates that the patient has a rheumatoid factor-positive condition, and is associated with a poor prognosis.

Investigations

There is often a mild normochromic normocytic anaemia. The erythrocyte sedimentation rate (ESR) is elevated, as is the level of C-reactive protein, during acute episodes of inflammation of the joints. The main diagnostic test is the detection of rheumatoid factor in the blood. Aspiration of synovial fluid shows the presence of increased levels of protein, a slight reduction in glucose concentration, and polymorphonuclear leucocytes present in the fluid.

The diagnosis is based on the presence of four or more of the following criteria:

1 hand involvement in an inflammatory arthritis

2 symmetrical joint involvement

3 arthritis of three or more joints that lasts for six or more weeks

4 morning stiffness

5 the presence of rheumatoid factor

6 the presence of rheumatoid nodules

7 the presence of erosions on X-ray of the small joints of the hands and/or feet.

Treatment

In the early stages, during the acute inflammatory process, the patient should be advised to rest their joints, and this sometimes involves splinting the joints. The specific drug therapy is described below.

Analgesics

Analgesics are given in the form of either simple paracetamol or more commonly non-steroidal anti-inflammatory drugs, which not only reduce the pain and discomfort but are also effective in reducing the inflammatory process.

Disease-modifying drugs

These drugs are designed to suppress or modulate the autoimmune process. They do not have an immediate therapeutic effect, and up to 4–6 months of treatment may be necessary to obtain a full response. Drugs in this group include D-penicillamine, gold and antimalarial drugs such as hydroxychloroquine.

Steroid drugs

These drugs have a potent anti-inflammatory action, and are generally used for patients whose condition is not well controlled by non-steroidal anti-inflammatory drugs, or in whom there is evidence of extra-articular involvement, such as neuropathy, renal disease or lung disease. Initially, high doses of steroids are used (eg prednisolone 60 mg daily). These doses are then gradually reduced while

CASE
78

monitoring the activity of the disease process and inflammatory markers such as ESR and C-reactive protein.

Immunosuppressive drugs

These drugs are used to suppress rheumatoid factor production and thus reduce the circulating levels of the immune complexes that cause the inflammatory reaction to occur. This group of drug includes methotrexate, azathioprine and cyclophosphamide.

Specific anticytokine drugs

With the development of agents that can inhibit the actions of interleukins and tumour necrosis factor, a number of drugs are now available that inhibit the cytokines which trigger the inflammatory reaction in this condition. Monoclonal antibodies and recombinant DNA technology have resulted in the development of a whole range of drugs which can inhibit the action of cytokines or block the receptors to which they normally attach. The potential for the use of these drugs in suppressing the disease activity of rheumatoid arthritis has been demonstrated. However, the potential for increasing the risk of infection and the development of malignancy as a consequence of long-term therapy must also be considered.

Musculoskeletal disorders

CASE 78

Musculoskeletal disorders

CASE 79

Systemic sclerosis (scleroderma)

This condition may be encountered at a clinical station or at a station showing a photograph of a patient with a characteristic appearance of the face or hands.

Definition

Systemic sclerosis is a connective tissue disorder in which there is vascular occlusion or insufficiency and the laying down of fibrous tissue in multiple organs and tissues. It is three times more common in women than in men, and the usual age of onset is 30–50 years.

Clinical features

Scleroderma is a progressive disorder that often presents with thickening of the skin and subcutaneous tissues and impaired blood flow, particularly to the peripheries. Patients usually describe symptoms of Raynaud's phenomenon affecting the fingers and toes. They may have difficulty swallowing, due to involvement of the blood vessels of the oesophagus and oesophageal immotility, and they may develop shortness of breath as a result of pulmonary fibrosis and pulmonary hypertension. On clinical examination there is thickening and binding down of the skin with acrosclerosis, loss of skin creases in the fingers and toes, poor circulation, telangiectasia and a typical facial appearance. There is loss of skin creases on the forehead, tethering of the skin over the nose and cheeks, and the skin of the face around the mouth becomes affected. The mouth can get progressively smaller in size, and this symptom can be so severe that the patient finds it increasingly difficult to open their mouth wide enough to eat. Involvement of the lacrimal and salivary glands can result in Sjögren's syndrome.

CREST syndrome

A variant of systemic sclerosis is CREST syndrome – CREST stands for **C**alcinosis, **R**aynaud's phenomenon, o**E**sophageal dysfunction, **S**clerodactyly and **T**elangiectasia. These patients have a very characteristic constellation of features, and X-ray of the hands may show evidence of subcutaneous calcification.

CASE 79

Investigations

There may be a mild normochromic normocytic anaemia and a raised erythrocyte sedimentation rate (ESR). Around 30% of patients will be rheumatoid factor-positive and 30–50% may show elevated levels of gammaglobulin. X-rays show evidence of subcutaneous atrophy with or without calcinosis. There may be features of resorption of the terminal phalanges. If pulmonary fibrosis is present, the chest X-ray will show evidence of mid- or lower-zone fibrotic change.

Treatment and management

There is no specific treatment for this condition. The patient should be advised to try to prevent injury to the hands, and to protect their hands and feet from cold temperatures and trauma. Symptoms of reflux oesophagitis should be treated with antacids or drugs that inhibit gastric acid production. Pulmonary fibrosis, if it occurs, usually progresses, and although steroids and immunosuppressive drugs have been tried there is no evidence that they are of any significant benefit. The only possibility of cure for this complication is by lung transplant.

Musculoskeletal disorders

Musculoskeletal disorders

CASE 80

Systemic lupus erythematosus (SLE)

This condition affects 1 in 1000 of the population worldwide, and is approximately ten times more common in women than in men. It is a serious disorder which can be encountered in the OSCE examination as part of a clinical examination station or a data interpretation station.

Definition

SLE is an immune complex disorder in which autoantibody is produced against nuclear material of the patient, and circulating immune complexes form which are precipitated in small blood vessels, causing vasculitis. Although this can affect any tissue or organ, it predominantly affects skin, synovial tissues of joints and the kidneys. It is characterised by periods of remission and relapse, and usually affects young women, with an onset at age 20–30 years.

Clinical features

Patients usually present with features of skin rash, which characteristically has a 'butterfly' distribution over the bridge of the nose and cheeks, and an inflammatory arthritis that usually affects the small joints of the hands and feet, and which causes pain, swelling and stiffness of the joints, but unlike rheumatoid arthritis does not result in lasting deformity of the joint. The patient may have constitutional symptoms of fever, weight loss and general malaise.

The vasculitic process may affect any tissue or organ, and although skin rash, joint pain and renal disease are characteristic, other manifestations include inflammation of blood vessels in the pleura causing pleuritic chest pains and pleural effusion, inflammation of the pericardium causing symptoms of pericarditis, or organic neurological conditions due to vasculitis in the central nervous system.

If left untreated, 50% of patients will develop inflammation of the small vessels of the glomerulus, resulting in acute or chronic renal impairment.

Investigations

Antinuclear antibody and double-stranded DNA antibodies, although not always present, are highly specific for this condition. The patient may have a normochromic

CASE 80

normocytic anaemia and a raised erythrocyte sedimentation rate (ESR) during episodes of inflammation. Characteristically, the level of C-reactive protein is **not** elevated during acute relapses of the condition. Rheumatoid factor may be positive, and the patient may have a false-positive serological test for syphilis. Antibodies against platelets and white blood cells can cause thrombocytopenia and neutropenia, respectively.

The diagnosis is made if four or more of the following features are present at any time during the course of the illness:

1 butterfly rash

2 discoid lupus rash

3 Raynaud's phenomenon

4 alopecia

5 photosensitivity skin rash

6 oral ulceration

7 a non-deforming arthritis

8 a false-positive test for syphilis

9 presence of antinuclear antibodies

10 evidence of renal involvement (eg proteinuria or reduced glomerular filtration rate)

11 serositis (ie pleurisy, pericarditis or peritonitis)

12 evidence of neurological involvement (eg the presence of convulsions, a psychotic condition or an organic brain syndrome)

13 evidence of a haematological disorder (eg thrombocytopenia or leucopenia)

14 an immunological abnormality consistent with the condition (eg the presence of circulating immune complexes, a positive double-stranded DNA antibody or antibodies to extractable nuclear antigens, hypocomplementaemia).

Patients with SLE must be carefully investigated for evidence of major organ involvement, especially renal disease, which is the commonest cause of death in these individuals.

Treatment

Treatment is based on analgesia for the joint pain, and in particular the use of non-steroidal anti-inflammatory drugs. If there is evidence of major organ involvement, steroids at high dose and immunosuppressive drugs such as cyclophosphamide or azathioprine are used to bring the disease under control, to reduce the inflammatory reaction and to suppress autoantibody production. Once the condition is under control

Musculoskeletal disorders

CASE 80

the dose of these drugs can be reduced and disease activity monitored by means of the ESR, the level of antinuclear antibody and double-stranded DNA antibody and the clinical features.

It is therefore important that renal function is regularly assessed using 24-hour urine collections and blood sampling for protein excretion and creatinine clearance. Any evidence of renal inflammation should be promptly treated and the patient's condition carefully monitored.

CASE 80

CASE 81

Paget's disease of bone

This condition may be encountered at a clinical station with a real patient displaying features of Paget's disease, at an X-ray station or at a data interpretation station where the student is given the biochemical profile of a patient with abnormal bone data.

Definition

Paget's disease is a chronic progressive disorder of bone in which normal structure is replaced by chemically abnormal bone. The condition is rare in individuals under the age of 30 years, and its incidence increases with age. It is twice as common in men than in women, and there tends to be a positive family history in patients who are affected.

Clinical features

The condition is usually asymptomatic, but there is a slowly progressive resorption of normal bone and replacement with abnormal bone which shows enlarged trabeculae and some deformity. During disease activity the abnormal bone may feel warm to the touch as a result of increased vascularity, and the patient may describe bone pain. There is an increased risk of pathological or stress fracture. Involvement of the skull results in enlargement of the head, and the patient may describe headache or symptoms caused by damage to cranial nerves. Deafness is common due to compression of the auditory nerve. Spinal involvement can result in kyphosis.

Investigations

The classic biochemical profile of these patients consists of normal serum calcium and phosphate levels, but markedly elevated alkaline phosphatase activity (more than ten times normal). The amount of calcium excreted in the urine is characteristically increased, and this can result in the formation of renal calculi.

X-ray of the skull shows increased thickness of the bones of the vault. Other bones show an increase in bone density, and flame-shaped lucid areas may be apparent.

Treatment

The mainstay of treatment is the use of bisphosphonates to prevent weakening of the bones, and analgesics to relieve the pain.

CASE
81

Musculoskeletal disorders

CASE 82

Osteoporosis

This condition is most commonly seen at a radiology station, usually with an X-ray of the spine showing the classic features of the disorder.

📖 Definition

Osteoporosis is defined as a decrease in the quantity of bone per unit volume. The bone is normal both histologically and in chemical composition.

? Causes

The main causes of osteoporosis are as follows:

1 **Hormonal causes.** This condition most commonly occurs in post-menopausal women.

2 **Disuse osteoporosis.** The skeleton can become osteoporotic as a result of immobilisation or loss of function. The condition can therefore be seen in patients who are bedbound or who have neurological disease (eg motor neurone disease, poliomyelitis, Guillain-Barré syndrome).

3 **Nutritional causes.** Bones may become osteoporotic as a result of general protein and calcium malabsorption.

4 **Endocrine causes.** A number of endocrine abnormalities can result in generalised osteoporosis, in particular thyrotoxicosis and Cushing's syndrome.

5 **Causes associated with multiple myeloma.** Although multiple myeloma characteristically causes lytic lesions in bones, it may give rise to an appearance that is indistinguishable from generalised osteoporosis.

6 **Idiopathic.** Osteoporosis sometimes occurs in young people with no obvious underlying cause. In such cases it usually affects adolescents or pregnant women and is characterised by severe bone pain.

CASE 82

Clinical features

If osteoporosis is a result of any of the conditions mentioned above, the clinical features of those disorders will also be present. In the commonest form of osteoporosis (ie post-menopausal), the symptoms usually appear after the age of 50 years. This condition affects approximately 25% of post-menopausal women. Involvement of the spine results in kyphosis, with loss of height, and the patient may complain of back pain and be susceptible to fractures, especially of the vertebral column or neck of femur.

Investigations

Characteristically, the X-ray shows thinning of the bone, with maintenance of calcium outlining the periphery of the bone. This is particularly clearly seen on X-ray of the spinal column, and the appearance is termed 'pencilling'. The other characteristic features are loss of cortical thickness of bone, fewer trabeculae and decreased bone density. Pathological or stress fractures can sometimes be visualised, and wedge-shaped compression fractures of thoracic or lumbar vertebrae are common.

Treatment

The underlying cause, if present, should be treated. Patients require analgesics for bone pain, and prevention of further osteoporotic change is achieved by means of oestrogens in the form of hormone replacement therapy, a high-calcium diet or calcium supplementation together with bisphosphonates, which increase mineralisation of the bones.

Musculoskeletal disorders

CASE
82

Musculoskeletal disorders

CASE 83

Osteomalacia

This is an uncommon condition, although it can be encountered at a radiology station where X-rays with the classic features of this deficiency disorder may be shown, or at a data interpretation station, where the student is presented with a biochemical profile showing altered calcium levels.

Definition

Osteomalacia is defined as demineralisation or softening of bone due to deficiency of vitamin D or calcium.

Clinical features

This condition usually occurs in patients who suffer from malabsorption, and will therefore have the classic clinical features of this condition (see Case 34). In addition, patients often develop bone pain which is worse on weight-bearing. They may have tenderness of the bone or intermittent acute pain in weight-bearing bones due to the development of fractures or pseudofractures. The calcium deficiency results in proximal muscle weakness, and patients often describe difficulty in standing up from a sitting position, or in climbing stairs. Because of the proximal muscle weakness, the patient may exhibit a waddling gait. If there is significant hypocalcaemia, symptoms of carpopedal spasm or tetany may be present.

Investigations

X-rays of bones may show bowing or plastic deformity of the bone. The characteristic features are Looser's zones, which are pseudofractures (horizontal areas of radiolucency which run perpendicular to the free bone surface). They are often bilateral and symmetrical, and are best seen on the axillary border of the scapula, the femoral neck, the ischial tuberosity, the pubic rami or the ribs. Biochemical analysis shows a low calcium–phosphate product. The serum calcium and phosphate levels are reduced, alkaline phosphatase activity is increased and the urinary calcium excretion rate is decreased.

CASE
83

Treatment

Therapy is aimed at treatment of the underlying cause, together with calcium and vitamin D supplementation. Vitamin D intake should be increased by more than 1000 international units per day, together with calcium supplementation in the diet or the oral use of calcium salts.

Musculoskeletal disorders

CASE 83

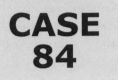

CASE 84

Gout

This deforming arthropathy can be mistaken for rheumatoid arthritis, and is often seen as part of a clinical station in OSCE examinations.

Definition and types

Gout is a disorder of uric acid metabolism that results in crystallisation of uric acid within the synovial fluid, causing an inflammatory arthritis.

Primary gout is an inherited disorder of purine metabolism, and 50–80% of patients have a positive family history.

Secondary gout is a disorder in which there are increased uric acid levels in the serum due to increased cell turnover. This condition may occur in polycythaemia, myelofibrosis, leukaemia or multiple myeloma, or as a result of rapid weight loss, cytotoxic drug therapy or other drugs (especially diuretics, which can increase serum urate levels).

Clinical features

The commonest form of presentation is with acute pain, swelling and inflammation of the first metatarsophalangeal joint of the foot. The patient may have constitutional symptoms of fever, sweating, loss of appetite and general malaise. Gouty arthritis may then affect several other joints and can present as a generalised polyarticular disorder. Uric acid may be precipitated not only in synovial fluid but also in periarticular tissues and cartilage (gouty tophi). The condition can be complicated by progressive renal failure and hypertension as a result of uric acid deposition in the kidneys, and renal stones (urate stones) may cause symptoms of renal colic. X-ray fails to show these stones because they are radiolucent.

Investigations

The patient characteristically has a raised serum urate level, a high erythrocyte sedimentation rate (ESR), and polymorphonuclear leucocytosis during episodes of acute inflammation.

CASE
84

Treatment

Acute attacks are treated with non-steroidal anti-inflammatory drugs or colchicine. Chronic gout is treated with drugs such as probenecid that increase uric acid excretion and therefore decrease the serum urate level. This treatment decreases the frequency and duration of attacks and reduces the risk of renal damage.

Inhibition of xanthine oxidase reduces the breakdown of purines and the formation of urate. This can be achieved by the use of allopurinol, 100 mg given three times daily, and this drug is often used as prophylaxis to prevent acute attacks.

It is important to remember that certain drugs can precipitate gout in a susceptible patient. These include the thiazide diuretics, furosemide (frusemide), acetazolamide and clofibrate.

Musculoskeletal disorders

CASE
84

Dermatology

CASE 85

Eczema

In OSCE examinations, this may be seen either as a clinical photograph or as a real patient with an itchy, excoriated skin rash.

Definition

Eczema is a chronic, relapsing, itchy skin rash that is often associated with other allergic disorders, especially asthma, allergic rhinitis and allergic conjunctivitis.

Clinical features

Approximately 80% of patients with atopic eczema have a personal or family history of allergic disease. The classic feature is an intensely itchy, erythematous rash with honey-coloured crusting which can occur on any region of the body, but most commonly affects the flexures, especially around the antecubital fossae, the popliteal fossae, the nape of the neck and behind the ears. The non-affected skin is usually dry, thickened and tends to lose water easily. The rash usually appears in infancy, and parents tend to associate its onset with weaning or changing from breastfeeding to cow's milk.

The rash is itchier in bed at night or if the patient is hot. Scratching also tends to exacerbate the rash, and can lead to a vicious cycle of rash, itching, scratching, worsening of the rash with increased itching, etc.

In most patients the condition tends to improve with age, and over 85% of cases will have completely resolved by the time they reach adolescence.

Treatment

1 **Skin hydration.** This is the key to good therapy. Emollients can be applied to the rash or added to bath water.

2 **Occlusive dressings.** For acute flare-ups of the rash and in order to break the cycle of scratching, itching and worsening rash, wet wraps containing agents to hydrate the skin can be used, and are highly effective.

3 **Topical steroids.** These are extremely effective in reducing the inflammatory reaction and itching. As a general rule, the lowest-potency

Dermatology

CASE 85

preparation that is effective for the patient should be used in order to reduce the risk of superimposed infection, thinning of the skin and systemic side effects. It is important that medium- or high-potency steroids are not used on the face, to avoid skin atrophy, depigmentation, capillary dilatation and acneform eruption.

4 **Antibiotics.** Superimposed infection should be treated with topical preparations containing an antibiotic-steroid combination. In cases of severe infection, systemic antibiotics are sometimes needed.

5 **Antigen avoidance measures.** Patients who have a definite history of exacerbation of their rash after eating certain foods, and who have a positive type I hypersensitivity test to food antigens, should be started on an elimination diet for a trial period. Many patients with atopic eczema are allergic to house-dust mite antigen. These patients often improve when strict house-dust mite antigen avoidance measures are instituted in their home.

CASE
85

CASE 86

Psoriasis

This condition may be shown in an OSCE examination as a clinical photograph of a patient with a skin rash or abnormal nails. It may also be encountered in a clinical examination station with a patient who has a skin rash, nail changes and joint disease.

Definition

Psoriasis is an inflammatory disorder that can affect the skin, the nails and the joints.

Clinical features

These can vary, both between patients and within an individual patient over the course of their illness.

Skin rash

This is the most frequently encountered manifestation of the disease. Well-demarcated red or pink erythematous plaques, which have adherent silvery-grey scales, form on the skin. The size of the skin plaques varies from small papules to large lesions, which can be annular or arcuate in shape with thick edges and an erythematous margin. Removal of scales can result in a punctate bleeding point at the site of detachment. The rash is not itchy and is most often present over extensor surfaces of the limbs, especially around the elbows and knees. Lesions occur on the scalp within the hairline, and may also occur in the areas of skin creases.

A variety of descriptive terms are used for psoriasis, usually related to the size of the skin lesions. They include the following:

- plaque – larger irregular-shaped lesions
- nummular – the size and shape of coins
- guttate (drop-like) – small papular lesions
- pustular – associated with pustules.

Dermatology

CASE 86

Nail changes

Psoriasis can and does affect other epithelial structures, especially the nail matrix and nail bed. There are four classic nail changes which may occur:

1 pitting – due to parakeratosis in the nail plate as the nail grows out from under the nail fold

2 grease spots – due to involvement of the mid-portion of the nail matrix by the inflammatory process

3 onycholysis – distal separation of the nail plate from the nail bed occurs as a result of proliferation of the epithelium in the nail bed

4 nail dystrophy – the nail plate may be diffusely affected and result in nail dystrophy.

Joint disease

This affects 5% of patients with psoriasis. The patient develops an inflammatory arthritis which is often asymmetrical and commonly affects the interphalangeal (IP) joints of the fingers and/or toes, resulting in 'sausage digits', but can be symmetrical and localised to the distal IP joints only. Larger joints may be affected, and the sacroiliac joints are commonly involved.

Over 75% of patients with joint disease will show associated nail changes. Rheumatoid factor is negative, but the serum urate level may be increased due to the rapid turnover of epithelial cells. X-ray will show a destructive arthritis with resorption of bone around the affected joints, and there may be telescoping of the digits (arthritis mutilans).

Treatment

Skin disease

1 **Lubricants.** These reduce the risk of fissure formation within plaques and maintain the flexibility of the surrounding skin.

2 **Coal tar preparations.** These have a definite effect in reducing inflammation and cell turnover in plaques. There are problems with staining of skin, irritant properties and odour, which can be reduced by using extracts or refined products.

3 **Topical steroids.** These are highly effective treatments, but excessive use can cause skin thinning or even systemic side effects.

**CASE
86**

4 **Phototherapy.** Ultraviolet radiation either alone or combined with photosensitising drugs is the main treatment used for patients with severe skin disease and for those cases that are resistant to conventional drug therapy. The psoralen compounds are used as photosensitising agents together with ultraviolet A irradiation (a treatment known as PUVA therapy).

5 **Systemic drugs.** A number of drugs can be used to reduce the rate of skin cell turnover or to alter the inflammatory reaction. These include:

- methotrexate – a cytotoxic drug
- retinoids (synthetic analogues of vitamin A)
- ciclosporin – this drug modulates the cell-mediated immune system and has been shown to be effective in reducing inflammation in psoriasis.

Joint disease

1 Supportive therapy – joint splints during episodes of disease activity.

2 Anti-inflammatory analgesics – using non-steroidal anti-inflammatory drugs.

3 Intra-articular steroid injection – for episodes of acute inflammation.

4 Physiotherapy – to maintain the full range of movement.

Dermatology

CASE
86

CASE 87

Erythema nodosum

This condition is often encountered at an OSCE station as a clinical photograph which is shown to the student to test both their ability to recognise the typical skin lesions and their knowledge of the underlying causes.

Definition

Erythema nodosum is an erythematous nodular eruption which is painful, tender, and often occurs over the shins.

? Causes

Erythema nodosum may occur as a primary disorder with no obvious underlying cause, but more commonly it is secondary to some underlying condition. It behaves like an immune complex disorder, and predominantly affects the blood vessels of the skin on the exterior aspects of the lower legs.

If erythema nodosum is not a primary disorder, it may be secondary to any of the following conditions:

1 Infection:
- post-streptococcal
- tuberculosis
- cat scratch fever
- fungal infection.

2 Neoplasia:
- lymphoma or leukaemia.

3 Drugs:
- sulphonamides
- oral contraceptive pill.

CASE
87

4 Inflammatory disease:

- sarcoidosis
- Crohn's disease
- ulcerative colitis.

Clinical features

The patient develops painful red raised lesions on the shins, which usually appear and resolve within a period of 4–6 weeks. Less commonly the extensor aspects of the lower arms may be affected. Constitutional symptoms of malaise and fever often occur. The patient may have a history of previous infection, such as streptococcal sore throat 7–10 days previously, or a history of inflammatory bowel disease, sarcoidosis or drug therapy.

The lesions feel hot to the touch and are tender. Some lesions heal while new ones may form, but generally they all eventually resolve without any residual scarring.

Investigations

The patient should be carefully investigated to identify any underlying cause. Investigations should include a chest X-ray to look for evidence of tuberculosis or sarcoidosis, a throat swab and blood sample for ASO titre to rule out current or recent streptococcal infection, and a full blood picture, total and differential white cell count and serum immunoglobulins to rule out leukaemia or lymphoma. If the patient has any gastrointestinal symptoms, barium contrast studies of large and small bowel, together with inflammatory markers (erythrocyte sedimentation rate (ESR) and C-reactive protein) should be undertaken to investigate possible inflammatory bowel disease.

Treatment

1 Treat the underlying cause if possible.
2 Bedrest – patients with this condition recover more quickly and with less risk of relapse if they have strict bedrest.
3 Analgesia – non-steroidal anti-inflammatory drugs are extremely effective in reducing the pain.
4 Steroids – prednisolone should only be used to treat severe or recurrent attacks that cannot be controlled by strict bedrest and analgesics.

Dermatology

CASE
87

CASE 88

Neurofibromatosis

This condition may be encountered in the OSCE examination either as a clinical photograph showing multiple skin lesions, or as a real patient with skin lesions at a clinical examination station.

Definition

Neurofibromatosis is an inherited condition (usually autosomal dominant) in which tumours develop on the nerves of the skin and internal organs.

Clinical features

The patient will usually have a positive family history of the condition. During the course of their life they develop multiple flesh-coloured skin lesions which are dome-shaped and can be easily pressed into the skin and/or subcutaneous nodules which are neurofibromas of subcutaneous nerves. They also display café-au-lait skin lesions (present in more than 90% of cases), and may have multiple pigmented naevi or freckles. Neurofibromas develop on nerves to internal organs, and may develop in the central nervous system, which can result in learning disability. Lesions in bone can result in bone cysts, while fibromas of the gastrointestinal tract may cause intestinal bleeding or obstruction. Patients with neurofibromatosis have an increased incidence of acoustic neuroma, phaeochromocytoma and coarctation of the aorta.

Approximately 10–15% of patients will develop a sarcomatous (malignant) change in one or more of the neurofibromas.

Treatment

1   Genetic counselling is important, to inform the patient of the mode of inheritance and to advise them that any children they may have will almost certainly be affected.

2   If any of the complications listed above arise, they should be treated. Surgical treatment may sometimes be necessary for intestinal bleeding or obstruction or for removal of tumours that are causing pressure effects or are malignant.

CASE 88

CASE 89

Skin cancers

Students are expected to be able to recognise the three main types of malignancy that occur in the skin. At an OSCE station these may appear together as a series of clinical photographs of skin lesions.

 ## Definitions

There are three main types of skin cancer:

1 squamous-cell carcinoma

2 basal-cell carcinoma

3 malignant melanoma.

Squamous-cell carcinoma

This is a malignant tumour that arises from the squamous epithelium of the skin. It occurs more commonly in the elderly, usually on sun-exposed skin. It is also more common in patients who are immunosuppressed (eg renal transplant patients).

Clinical features

The patient develops a hyperkeratotic, crusting lesion, which will usually slowly enlarge and ulcerate. It occurs on sun-exposed skin, and other precancerous hyperkeratotic lesions may be found, especially on the face, scalp and ears. Squamous-cell carcinoma may occur on the lip, especially in pipe smokers, as a result of exposure to carcinogens in tobacco tar.

The lesion becomes a spreading, invasive ulcer, but may present as a rapidly growing nodule. The cancer is locally destructive and can spread to local lymph nodes or via the bloodstream to other organs.

Treatment

In the early stages excision is curative, while larger lesions may require radiotherapy. If regional lymph nodes are enlarged these should be removed, and distant spread may require systemic chemotherapy.

CASE 89

Dermatology

Basal-cell carcinoma

This is the commonest of all skin cancers, and it is a common neoplasm of the skin of the face. It never metastasises, grows slowly but can invade deeply, and may recur after treatment.

Clinical features

Basal-cell lesions develop on the skin of the face above a line between the angle of the mouth and the external auditory meatus, commonly on the side of the nose or around the eye. They develop as pearly, flesh-coloured or translucent papules or nodules with rolled edges. Telangiectatic blood vessels are often present over the surface of the lesion. The centre becomes necrotic, ulcerates and becomes crusted as the lesion enlarges.

Basal-cell tumours do not spread to regional nodes or via the bloodstream, and are only life-threatening if they spread locally to invade underlying tissues such as bone, sinuses or blood vessels.

Treatment

Small lesions can be treated by means of cryosurgery, curettage or cautery. Large lesions may require radiotherapy or surgical excision together with skin grafting. Recurrence occurs after treatment in 10–20% of lesions.

Malignant melanoma

This is a highly malignant skin tumour derived from melanocytes which spreads via lymphatics and the bloodstream. The incidence of this skin cancer in the UK is increasing at a rate of 100% every 10 years. Risk factors include the following:

- excessive sun exposure, especially in childhood
- family history of melanoma
- fair skin
- multiple pigmented naevi.

Clinical features

The patient may notice a pigmented lesion which starts to change in appearance, enlarge, become darker in colour or ulcerate. The development of itching in or bleeding from a pigmented naevus should also raise concern that a malignant transformation has occurred. The appearance may be that of a superficial spreading pigmented lesion or a pigmented nodule. In men, lesions most often occur on the back, while in women the leg is the commonest site.

CASE
89

Because of the early spread of these lesions, any suspicious pigmented lesion should be biopsied.

Treatment

Wide and deep excision of the primary lesion is essential. If regional lymph nodes are enlarged, these should be excised and the patient regularly followed up to look for evidence of local, regional or distant recurrence. Chemotherapy and immunotherapy are best planned at specialist clinics.

Occasionally patients may present with secondary tumours and little to find on examination of the skin.

The prognosis will depend on the size of the primary tumour, the degree of spread and the duration of disease.

Dermatology

CASE
89

Renal disorders

CASE 90

Acute renal failure

It is of vital importance that junior doctors have a knowledge of the causes, early signs and treatment of acute renal failure. This acute medical emergency often appears in the OSCE examination as a data interpretation station (with a fluid balance chart, blood pressure record chart or biochemical profile), or in a station that is testing knowledge of therapeutics and pharmacology (treatment of hyperkalaemia).

Definition

Acute renal failure is a sudden failure of the kidneys to excrete toxic waste products and control fluid, electrolyte and acid–base balance.

? Causes

There are three types of acute renal failure, namely pre-renal, renal and post-renal.

Pre-renal type

The common factor is hypotension. If the systolic pressure falls below 80 mmHg and remains low for more than 2–3 hours, renal perfusion will shut down in order to preserve cerebral blood pressure. If there is no perfusion of the kidneys, renal function will come to an abrupt halt and the features of acute renal failure will develop.

The common causes of pre-renal renal failure are as follows:

- myocardial infarction (reduced systolic pressure)
- haemorrhage (hypovolaemia)
- severe burns (hypovolaemia)
- septicaemia (vasodilatation)
- cardiac arrhythmia (reduced systolic pressure)
- hepatorenal syndrome.

Renal disorders

CASE
90

Renal type

Any disease process that affects both kidneys, impairing their ability to filter, resorb or excrete urine, will cause a sudden onset of the features of the renal type of acute renal failure. These precipitating conditions include the following:

- acute glomerulonephritis
- renal papillary necrosis
- acute interstitial nephritis (drug-induced)
- renal vessel vasculitis
- acute pyelonephritis.

There is considerable reserve renal tissue – indeed, patients can function with less than a quarter of one kidney (ie less than an eighth of their total renal function; see assessment of renal function below). Therefore any condition that causes acute renal failure must affect the kidneys to such an extent that the damage is extensive and bilateral.

Post-renal type

For the reasons mentioned in the previous paragraph, acute renal failure will only develop if there is obstruction to the outflow of **both** kidneys. Conditions which cause this include the following:

1 Obstruction of both ureters:
- retroperitoneal tumour
- retroperitoneal fibrosis.

2 Obstruction of the bladder outlet:
- carcinoma of the bladder
- bladder stone.

3 Obstruction of the urethra:
- benign prostatic hypertrophy
- prostatic carcinoma
- urethral stricture.

By far the commonest post-renal cause is prostatic enlargement in men.

CASE 90

📝 Clinical features

Whatever the cause, the first clinical feature is a reduction in urinary output, with a volume of less than 500 ml in 24 hours (oliguria) or no urine production in 24 hours (anuria). If the underlying cause is not corrected, the patient will develop features of fluid retention, electrolyte abnormalities, rising levels of urea and creatinine in the blood, and clinical features associated with the accumulation of toxic waste products. As the condition worsens there is a progression of symptoms as follows:

1 general malaise

2 nausea with or without vomiting

3 oedema

4 sallow complexion

5 uraemic fetor ('mousy' smell of breath)

6 uraemic frost (white crystals of urea develop on the skin as sweat dries)

7 muscle twitching

8 reduced level of consciousness

9 convulsions

10 Kussmaul breathing (due to acidosis)

11 Cheyne-Stokes respiration

12 respiratory arrest and death.

💊 Treatment

Treatment of the underlying cause

If possible, it is vital to identify and rapidly correct the underlying cause.

1 **Pre-renal type.** Increase the blood pressure using intravenous fluid infusion together with drugs that increase systolic pressure (positive inotropes). No patient should be left with a systolic pressure of less than 80 mmHg for more than 1 hour.

2 **Post-renal type.** If the bladder is distended, the obstruction is in the urethra or bladder outlet. This can normally be relieved by passing a urinary catheter – if not, a suprapubic catheter should be inserted. If the obstruction is retroperitoneal, surgical intervention is necessary to allow urine to flow down the ureters.

Renal disorders

CASE
90

3 **Renal type.** The treatment of renal causes depends on the nature of the
disease process that is causing the kidney damage.

Fluid balance

It is essential that accurate measurements of fluid input and loss are recorded, and
the quantity of fluid given to the patient should be adjusted to maintain hydration
without causing fluid overload.

As a general rule, the total amount of fluid given in any 24-hour period should be
equal to the total volume of fluid lost in the preceding 24 hours plus 500 ml to
correct for insensible loss (sweating, respiratory fluid loss, etc). This will maintain a
steady-state fluid balance. Each day the amount of fluid is calculated, based on the
previous day's urinary output and, if indicated, loss of other fluids (eg vomitus,
diarrhoea, surgical drainage fluid).

Failure to maintain proper fluid balance is very dangerous for the patient. If the
urinary output is less than 500 ml per day and the patient is allowed to drink freely
or is given intravenous fluids to the extent that their daily intake is more than 1 litre,
it will not be long before the fluid overload manifests itself as peripheral and
pulmonary oedema. The patient then develops very severe shortness of breath and
can literally drown due to the presence of too much water in their lungs.

Correction of electrolyte disorders

Regular biochemical investigations should be undertaken to measure the levels of
urea, creatinine and the common electrolytes. In acute renal failure the most
significant abnormality that can occur is hyperkalaemia. If the serum potassium
concentration rises above the normal range (3.5–5.0 mmol/litre), there is a risk of
sudden cardiac arrest. Two measures can be used to prevent the occurrence of this
potentially life-threatening problem:

1 the patient should be commenced on a low-potassium diet
2 all potassium supplements (oral drugs, additions to intravenous fluids, etc)
   should be avoided.

If a high level of potassium develops, it can be reduced by the use of an ion-
exchange resin such as Calcium Resonium^R given orally or as an enema.

If the potassium level is dangerously high, it can be rapidly reduced by exploiting the
fact that potassium ions can be made to move into cells along with glucose under the
action of insulin. By infusing 50 ml of 50% dextrose over a period of 1–2 hours and
giving 20 units of soluble insulin 30 minutes after the start of the infusion, the serum
potassium level can be reduced. This therapy can be repeated, but is of only

CASE
90

Renal disorders

temporary benefit. It is therefore mainly used to 'buy time' while a more definitive therapy (peritoneal dialysis or haemodialysis) is organised.

Prevention of symptoms of uraemia

Most of the toxins that build up are formed by the breakdown of nitrogenous material (ie protein). To prevent the development of symptoms of uraemia, the patient can be started on a low-protein diet, but to ensure that they do not develop weakness or muscle wasting, additional calories are provided by supplementation of the diet with carbohydrates.

Despite all of the above treatment measures, some patients require dialysis until their renal function recovers. Only in a minority of cases (usually due to irreversible renal disease) is long-term dialysis or renal transplantation needed.

Renal disorders

CASE
90

CASE 91

Chronic renal failure

There are many patients with chronic renal disease who are able and willing to be used for undergraduate examinations. This condition is frequently encountered as part of a clinical examination station, or as data from biochemical investigations at a data interpretation station.

Definition

Chronic renal failure is an abnormally low glomerular filtration rate that persists for more than three months, usually as a result of an irreversible disease process affecting the renal parenchyma.

? Causes

These include the following:

- glomerulonephritis (30%)
- interstitial nephritis (20%)
- hypertension (10%)
- polycystic renal disease (10%)
- diabetic nephropathy (10%)
- chronic pyelonephritis (5%)
- other renal disorders (5%)
- unknown (10%).

Clinical features

These develop insidiously as the levels of urea and other toxic waste products slowly increase. The main features are easily remembered by considering the features of defects of the normal functions of the kidneys:

1. Excretion of fluid and toxic waste:
    - general malaise – nausea and vomiting
    - lethargy

CASE
91

- sallow complexion
- fluid retention – periorbital oedema, leg oedema
- pulmonary oedema.

2 Erythropoietin production – normochromic normocytic anaemia.

3 Calcium metabolism – features of hypocalcaemia (osteomalacia) due to failure of the kidney to hydroxylate to 1-alphacholecalciferol.

4 Acid–base balance – when advanced, the development of acidosis results in an increase in the rate and depth of respiration (Kussmaul breathing) as the body tries to reduce the acidosis by 'blowing off' carbon dioxide.

In contrast to acute renal failure, because the accumulation of toxins occurs more slowly in chronic renal failure, the patient has time to compensate and the symptoms are better tolerated. However, the anaemia and bone changes are more often a feature. Patients usually pass relatively normal volumes of fluid, or may even have polyuria due to the inability of the diseased kidneys to concentrate the urine.

Treatment

1 Treat the underlying disease process if possible.

2 Prevent fluid overload – careful assessment of urinary volume is essential, and the patient's fluid intake should be controlled to prevent either dehydration or fluid overload.

3 Electrolyte balance – prevent hyperkalaemia by giving the patient a low-potassium diet. Correct other electrolyte deficiencies by using supplements if necessary.

4 Correct anaemia – use erythropoietin injections to replace the deficiency.

5 Maintain calcium balance – treat the patient with 1-α-cholecalciferol if there is evidence of hypocalcaemia.

6 Prevent uraemia – the use of low-protein diets can prevent or delay the development of symptoms of uraemia.

7 Correct hypertension – it is vitally important to maintain a normal blood pressure to prevent the vicious spiral of renal damage which causes hypertension that in turn leads to further renal damage.

If the above measures fail to halt the progression of renal impairment, dialysis (either peritoneal or haemodialysis) is necessary, the only cure being renal transplantation.

Renal disorders

CASE
91

Assessment of renal function

As mentioned earlier, humans can survive on less than a quarter of one kidney (ie less than an eighth of their total renal function). This means that patients may have significant renal disease before they develop symptoms or clinical signs or display biochemical abnormalities such as elevated urea or serum creatinine levels. Demonstration of renal disease can be achieved by means of urinalysis, microscopy or the creatinine clearance test.

Urinalysis

Testing the urine with dipsticks will usually show the presence of protein and/or blood in patients with renal disease. This simple procedure can be used as a screening test, and is often encountered in OSCE examinations.

Microscopy

In patients with any inflammatory process in the glomeruli or renal tubules, microscopy of the urine will show the presence of inflammatory cells (pus cells) or renal tubular cells and debris (casts).

Creatinine clearance test

This is by far the best non-invasive test for assessing renal function. It gives a measure of the glomerular filtration rate (GFR) – that is, the volume of blood filtered by the kidneys in one minute.

The normal GFR is 110 ml/minute. Any disease process that affects the glomerulus or tubules will cause a reduction in GFR, even before the increase in urea or creatinine concentrations in the blood.

The creatinine clearance test is performed by obtaining a full 24-hour volume of urine and taking a single blood sample during the same 24-hour period. The following are measured:

1 the volume of urine passed in 24 hours (V)

2 the concentration of creatinine in the urine (U)

3 the plasma creatinine concentration (P).

The creatinine clearance is calculated using the following formula:

$$\text{creatinine clearance} = \frac{U \times V}{P}$$

**CASE
91**

Renal disorders

Normally this is equivalent to the GFR, and serial measurements with the creatinine clearance test can be used to monitor patients with chronic renal failure to assess either the progression of disease or the response to therapy.

CASE
91

CASE 92

Polycystic renal disease

This condition is often encountered at a clinical examination station where the student is asked to examine the abdomen of a patient and expected to find enlarged irregular renal masses.

Definition

Polycystic renal disease is a genetic disorder associated with the formation of renal cortical cysts. It is most often an autosomal dominant condition with 100% penetrance, and it usually presents in adult life. The rare autosomal recessive form usually presents in infancy.

Clinical features

Because of its autosomal dominant form of inheritance there is usually a positive family history. The renal cysts may appear at any age, but usually appear in the late teenage years or early adulthood. Bleeding or infection may occur, and therefore painless haematuria, renal infection or hypertension can be presenting features. On examination of the abdomen, irregular enlarged kidneys are usually easily palpable.

As the cysts enlarge they compress normal renal tissue, and this leads to slowly progressive renal failure. Anaemia is not usually a significant feature, as the cysts commonly produce erythropoietin.

Cysts may occur in other organs. For example, 30% of patients will have cysts in the liver, and some may have pancreatic or splenic cysts. There is an increased risk of cerebral artery berry aneurysm, and rupture of one of these will result in subarachnoid haemorrhage.

Investigations

The best diagnostic test is ultrasound scan of the abdomen, which will demonstrate the bilateral polycystic kidneys.

Changes in blood urea and creatinine levels and the creatinine clearance test will reflect the degree of renal impairment. Urine testing will often show the presence of haematuria and proteinuria, and bacteriology may reveal a significant number of organisms.

CASE
92

Renal disorders

Treatment

There is no specific treatment for polycystic renal disease, but any hypertension, urinary infection or symptoms due to renal failure should be treated. If severe chronic renal failure occurs, dialysis or renal transplantation should be considered.

Patients and their children should be given genetic counselling informing them of the risks of further generations having this condition, as well as the very significant risk of renal failure and complications of hypertension, and possible subarachnoid haemorrhage.

Renal disorders

CASE
92

CASE 93

Nephrotic syndrome

This syndrome is associated with the presence of large amounts of protein in the urine, and it may be encountered at data interpretation stations where urine analyses and biochemical profiles are shown to students.

Definition

Nephrotic syndrome is characterised by marked proteinuria (> 3 g/24 hours), hypoalbuminaemia and oedema, and is invariably associated with hypercholesterolaemia.

? Causes

Any renal disorder that involves the loss of large amounts of protein in the urine can result in nephrotic syndrome. The common causes are as follows:

- glomerulonephritis
- systemic lupus erythematosus
- diabetic glomerulosclerosis
- amyloidosis
- Henoch-Schönlein purpura
- drugs (eg penicillamine, captopril)
- renal vein thrombosis.

Although all forms of glomerulonephritis can cause nephrotic syndrome, membranous glomerulonephritis is the type that most commonly causes the condition in adults, and minimal-change glomerulonephritis most commonly causes it in children.

Clinical features

Because of the heavy protein loss in the urine, the patient may notice that their urine is frothy. As the serum albumin level falls, peripheral and even central oedema will develop and the patient will notice a puffiness around the eyes which is often most obvious first thing in the morning. The patient shows neither elevation of the jugular

CASE 93

venous pressure nor features of pulmonary oedema, and it is important to determine this to rule out congestive cardiac failure. Features of the primary underlying disease (eg systemic lupus erythematosus or diabetes) may be present.

Investigations

Nephrotic syndrome is characterised by proteinuria of more than 3 g/24 hours and a serum albumin concentration of less than 30 g/litre. A raised cholesterol level is invariably present due to increased hepatic synthesis, which accompanies the increased production of albumin by the liver.

There will be biochemical features of renal impairment, such as a reduced creatinine clearance test and increased serum creatinine and urea levels, together with large quantities of protein in the urine on dipstick testing.

Other laboratory abnormalities may be present, consistent with the underlying disease or disorder that is causing the renal damage.

Treatment

Identification and treatment of the underlying cause usually result in reduction of the proteinuria and correction of the nephrotic syndrome.

Oedema can be reduced by the careful use of thiazide or low-dose loop diuretics. In some cases albumin infusion may be helpful, but the benefit is only transient unless the protein loss can be stopped.

Renal disorders

CASE
93

CASE 94

Pyelonephritis

This could be encountered in a procedure station where the student is asked to dipstick test the urine, which contains a significant quantity of protein and possibly a trace of blood.

Definition and types

Pyelonephritis is infection (commonly bacterial) of the renal system, usually developing as a result of ascending infection.

Pyelonephritis may be acute or chronic:

1 acute – infection of the kidney or renal tract without evidence of renal impairment

2 chronic (reflux nephropathy) – usually a result of congenital failure of the ureterovesical sphincter to prevent reflux of urine back up the ureters during micturition. Recurrent infective episodes cause inflammation of the renal parenchyma with subsequent scarrings and renal impairment.

Clinical features

The patient develops fever, dysuria and frequency of micturition (needing to pass urine often, but only small volumes being passed). Severe infection may be associated with rigors (uncontrollable shivering).

The urine will be dark in colour and have a strong ammoniacal odour. It may appear cloudy or 'smoky' if it contains some red cells, or there may be frank haematuria. Pain in the loin together with acute tenderness in the renal angle is common.

Urine testing will show the presence of protein and blood, and on microscopy red blood cells and white cells (pus cells) will be evident. Urine culture will show a significant growth of organisms.

Renal disorders

CASE
94

In most cases (80%) of acute pyelonephritis the causative organism is *Escherichia coli* derived from the patient's bowel flora. Other organisms which may be responsible include *Proteus* species (10%), *Streptococcus faecalis* (5%), *Staphylococcus epidermidis* or other coliforms.

In chronic pyelonephritis a mixture of pathogenic organisms may be cultured from the urine, or with different episodes of infection different organisms may be responsible, but invariably they are coliforms.

With recurrent infective episodes, progressive renal damage occurs, the kidneys become scarred and shrunken and features of renal impairment develop.

Investigations

During acute infection the white cell count is elevated, with polymorphonuclear leucocytosis. The erythrocyte sedimentation rate (ESR) and C-reactive protein are elevated.

Urine culture usually reveals the causative organism(s) unless the urine sample is taken after antibiotic therapy has been initiated.

A micturating cystogram may show evidence of ureteric reflux of urine. Ultrasound scanning of the abdomen can be used to identify small, scarred kidneys in patients with chronic pyelonephritis.

In these patients biochemical analyses will show evidence of raised urea and creatinine levels if significant renal damage has occurred. Less severe disease will be detected by creatinine clearance testing.

Treatment

Antibiotic therapy should be commenced after midstream samples of urine have been collected for bacterial culture so that their antibiotic sensitivity can be determined.

Most cases respond to broad-spectrum penicillin antibiotics or trimethoprim. During acute or severe infection, intravenous penicillins or cephalosporins may be needed. In patients with chronic pyelonephritis, antibiotic therapy should be initiated promptly to prevent further renal damage, and in some cases long-term prophylactic antibiotic therapy may be required.

Renal disorders

CASE
94

Immunology

CASE 95

Anaphylactic shock

This is an acute medical emergency, and all doctors should be capable of recognising and treating it. It may be encountered as a must-pass station in an OSCE examination.

Definition

Anaphylactic shock is a type I IgE-mediated hypersensitivity reaction that occurs in allergic individuals in whom an antigen to which they have been sensitised is introduced into the circulation, causing widespread mast-cell degranulation.

Clinical features

This condition may be triggered by insect bites, stings with wasp or bee venom, injection of drugs or ingestion of foods to which the individual is allergic. The presence of an antigen in the bloodstream causes mast-cell degranulation, which results in the following symptoms:

- angio-oedema – soft tissue swelling which may affect any part of the body, but most often affects the soft tissues of the lips, tongue and periorbital region
- urticaria – the patient may develop an urticarial (nettle sting-like) skin rash or generalised erythematous lesions which are intensely itchy
- laryngeal oedema – soft tissue swelling of the larynx may cause obstruction of the upper airway. The patient develops stridor and then becomes distressed
- bronchospasm – mast cell-mediator release in the lower respiratory tract causes smooth muscle contraction in the airways. The patient develops shortness of breath, tachycardia and wheeze
- hypotension – mast-cell degranulation results in the release of mediators which cause vasodilatation, and a rapid fall in blood pressure may occur.

Immunology

CASE
95

Treatment

Urgent treatment is required for patients who have laryngeal oedema or hypotension. For adults:

1   0.5 ml of 1 in 1000 adrenaline (epinephrine) should be given intramuscularly immediately to reverse the anaphylactic shock. If the blood pressure does not improve, a further 0.5 ml can be given after 5 minutes.
2   100% oxygen should be administered by inhalation.
3   10–30 mg of the antihistamine chlorpheniramine should be given by slow intravenous injection.
4   Hydrocortisone 250 mg can be given intravenously – this will have little effect on the early phase of anaphylaxis, but will prevent or reduce the severity of the late-phase reaction.

Patients invariably respond to this medication within minutes. Over the subsequent 24–48 hours further doses of antihistamine and hydrocortisone can be given. The patient's pulse, blood pressure and respiratory rate should be checked frequently.

Any drug or food substance that may have triggered the reaction should be identified and repeat exposure avoided.

Immunology

CASE
95

CASE 96

Angio-oedema and urticaria

These disorders, which often occur together in a patient, may be encountered at OSCE stations where the student is shown a clinical photograph of a patient with soft tissue swelling or a skin rash.

Definition

Angio-oedema and urticaria are conditions which result from transient leakage of plasma into the skin (urticaria) or subcutaneous tissue or submucosal tissues (angio-oedema), usually as a result of mast-cell degranulation.

? Causes

In over 80% of patients with angio-oedema or urticaria no underlying cause can be identified. This is termed idiopathic angio-oedema or urticaria. In 15–20% of cases the condition is secondary to some allergic reaction, or due to a physical or chemical stimulus that causes mast cells to become disrupted and release their chemical mediators.

The classification of causes of angio-oedema/urticaria is as follows:

1 idiopathic (80–85% of cases)
2 allergic – due to ingestion of a food antigen or drug (eg penicillin) to which the patient is sensitised
3 physical:
    - pressure
    - solar
    - cold
    - water
    - sweating (cholinergic).
4 chemical – due to ingestion of artificial colourings or preservatives in food or drinks. These chemical compounds directly activate mast cells
5 autoimmune:

Immunology

CASE 96

- associated with systemic lupus erythematosus
- hypocomplementaemic vasculitis.

6 hereditary angio-oedema – due to C1 esterase inhibitor deficiency.

7 drugs:

- non-steroidal anti-inflammatory drugs
- angiotensin-converting enzyme (ACE) inhibitors
- aspirin.

 # Clinical features

The patient suddenly develops episodes of soft tissue swelling which may affect any part of the body, but most commonly affect the soft tissues of the lips, tongue and periorbital region. The swelling (angio-oedema) may occur in isolation or be associated with an itchy, nettle sting-like skin rash (urticaria) which has a central weal with surrounding erythema, or the rash may consist of red erythematous blotches which occur on any part of the skin surface.

The swelling and individual skin lesions can last for up to 24 hours or more, and new lesions appear over a period of days.

In the idiopathic form of this condition there is no identifiable cause or triggering factor, and the patient may experience attacks either daily or infrequently over a period of many weeks or months.

If the condition is due to an allergy, a physical stimulus or a chemical additive, the patient can often identify the factor that precipitates an attack.

Hereditary angio-oedema (C1 esterase inhibitor deficiency)

This is the most severe form of the condition, which results from an autosomal dominant gene defect causing a deficiency of C1 esterase inhibitor in the blood. This substance is required to inhibit activation of the complement cascade. If complement activation occurs as a result of infection or trauma, severe angio-oedema of the skin and gastrointestinal tract will occur, which causes severe crampy abdominal pain or obstruction of the upper airway.

The patient usually has a strong family history of the condition, and there may be a family history of sudden death during or after surgery or dental extraction. Patients should not undergo either of these procedures without receiving fresh plasma or C1 esterase inhibitor concentrate to prevent life-threatening angio-oedema.

CASE
96

Investigations

To investigate the possibility of allergy as an underlying cause, a blood sample can be used to measure the serum IgE level and an allergy screening test performed (eg radioallergosorbent test, RAST) to identify antigen-specific IgE to food or drug antigens suspected as possible triggering factors.

C1 esterase inhibitor levels are extremely low or undetectable in patients with hereditary angio-oedema. Patients with hypocomplementaemic vasculitis have low complement levels during acute attacks, and anti-C1q antibodies can be detected in the serum.

Patients with chemical-induced angio-oedema will remain symptom-free if they adhere to a strict elimination diet avoiding artificial colourings and preservatives.

Treatment

If a drug or food antigen or additive is identified as a triggering factor, this should be eliminated from the diet. Similarly, if a physical cause is identified and avoided, the patient's condition will resolve.

For patients with idiopathic urticaria and angio-oedema, treatment with a non-sedating antihistamine is the only form of therapy that is available. These drugs can be used intermittently to abort acute attacks, or as regular daily medication to prevent attacks in patients who have frequent symptoms. Sometimes a combination of two or more antihistamines is required.

Steroids, although extremely effective for this condition, should not be used as routine treatment because of the risk of side effects. The vast majority of patients can be controlled with antihistamines.

The idiopathic form of this condition usually resolves spontaneously with time, but can persist for up to three years.

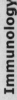

Immunology

CASE
96

CASE 97

Vasculitis

This topic seldom arises during an OSCE, but if it is encountered this will usually be at a data interpretation station, where a biochemical profile, antineutrophil cytoplasmic antibody test results, and sometimes urine analysis showing haematuria and proteinuria are presented to the student.

Definition

Vasculitis is defined as inflammation of blood vessels which occurs as a result of immune complex deposition and leads to vascular damage. The clinical features are determined by the type, size and location of the vessels involved.

Classification

Primary vasculitis

There is no underlying medical condition or 'foreign' antigen, such as a drug, which causes formation of the immune complex. Primary vasculitis is subclassified according to the size of the arteries involved:

- large (eg giant-cell arteritis) (see Case 100)
- medium (eg polyarteritis nodosa)
- small (eg Wegener's granulomatosis).

Secondary vasculitis

There is some underlying disease or exogenous antigen stimulating the formation of antigen–antibody complexes. Some of the commonest causes include the following:

- rheumatoid arthritis
- systemic lupus erythematosus
- inflammatory bowel disease
- subacute bacterial endocarditis
- drug-induced vasculitis (eg that induced by antibiotics).

Immunology

CASE 97

Polyarteritis nodosa

This is a relatively rare condition, but it is extremely important as it has a significant mortality rate if left untreated.

Clinical features

Polyarteritis nodosa is more common in men than in women, with a male:female ratio of 3:1. It can develop at any age, but more commonly occurs in older patients (50–60 years or older).

Non-specific symptoms of fever, malaise, general weakness, anorexia and weight loss are common. The other features depend on the site of blood vessel damage. Although the condition may affect any organ or tissue, it most commonly affects the blood vessels which supply the skin, gastrointestinal tract, joints and kidneys.

The patient may develop a widespread 'vasculitic' skin rash with areas of central necrosis, each of which is surrounded by an area of inflammation. Episodes of abdominal pain or gastrointestinal haemorrhage may occur, as can joint paint with swelling and inflammation. The most serious complication (which develops in 70% of patients) is renal vasculitis, which can cause hypertension and renal failure.

If this condition is not treated aggressively, there is a significant risk of acute renal failure and death. Involvement of coronary arteries can occur in polyarteritis nodosa, leading to myocardial infarction, heart failure or pericarditis.

Investigations

1 Full blood picture – this may show evidence of anaemia due to renal or gastrointestinal blood loss, and the total white cell count is usually elevated.

2 The erythrocyte sedimentation rate (ESR) is usually very high and the C-reactive protein level is raised.

3 Urine analysis – if renal arteries are affected, blood and protein will be detected in the urine. Creatinine clearance testing may show a reduced glomerular filtration rate.

4 Biochemical profile – this will show raised serum creatinine and urea levels if there is renal involvement.

5 Antineutrophil cytoplasmic antibody (ANCA) – in classic polyarteritis nodosa this test is negative. However, in a variant form of the disease (microvascular polyarteritis nodosa) the pANCA is often detected (cf Wegener's granulomatosis; see below).

Immunology

CASE
97

6   Radiology – contrast imaging of blood vessels (angiography) often reveals microaneurysms affecting medium-sized arteries, most commonly sited near the branching points of the vessels.

7   Skin biopsy – histological examination of a biopsy from a classic skin lesion will show perivascular inflammation of the dermal vessels with fibrinoid necrosis.

Treatment

The patient should initially be treated with high-dose corticosteroids (eg prednisolone 60 mg daily) in order to reduce the inflammatory process and prevent renal failure. Disease activity can be monitored by the constitutional symptoms, clinical signs, ESR and C-reactive protein level. Once the disease is under control the dosage of steroids can be reduced, but sometimes azathioprine is required as a steroid-sparing agent to keep the inflammatory reaction under control.

Wegener's granulomatosis

This is a form of primary vasculitis that affects small blood vessels and has a characteristic clinical pattern and highly specific and sensitive markers of disease activity. It causes necrotising granulomas to form in the respiratory tract, and is associated with crescentic glomerulonephritis, which has a high mortality rate.

Clinical features

The patient usually develops constitutional symptoms of fever, malaise, anorexia and weight loss, and often gives a history of chronic or recurrent sinusitis. Nasal crusting and nosebleeds are common, as the granulomatous vasculitis often affects the nasal mucosa. If the lower respiratory tract is involved, cough, pleuritic chest pains and haemoptysis are common symptoms. The patient may become extremely unwell, with fever, weight loss and respiratory symptoms that may give the clinical impression of an underlying lung tumour or tuberculosis.

In 80% of patients, vasculitis of the renal arteries results in a crescentic glomerulo-nephritis, which can lead to renal failure and, if not treated, is the main cause of death in patients with this disease.

Investigations

1   **ANCA test.** This is a very sensitive and specific test for this condition, and is positive in over 90% of patients. It is a fluorescent antibody test which in Wegener's granulomatosis shows a characteristic speckled staining pattern of

CASE 97

Immunology

the cytoplasm (cANCA). If a perinuclear staining pattern (pANCA) is seen, this is more consistent with the microvascular variant of polyarteritis, but it also occurs in systemic lupus erythematosus and inflammatory bowel disease.

2 **Renal function tests.** Analysis of urine will show the presence of blood and protein, and the creatinine clearance test will reveal a reduced glomerular filtration rate if renal vasculitis is present.

3 **Nasal biopsy.** Biopsy of the nasal mucosa will show evidence of a necrotising vasculitis with granuloma formation.

4 **Chest X-ray.** If the lower respiratory tract is involved, the chest X-ray will show areas of consolidation with cavity formation.

Treatment

Wegener's granulomatosis is usually controlled by the use of corticosteroids (prednisolone 60 mg daily), cyclophosphamide 4 mg/kg daily and co-trimoxazole 800 mg daily, with patients showing a dramatic improvement within 48–72 hours of starting therapy. Once the condition has been brought under control, the dose of therapy can be reduced. The effectiveness of drug therapy and evidence of disease activity correlate with the level of cANCA in the serum.

If left untreated this condition has a mortality rate of 90% within five years, but with therapy this is reduced to less than 5%.

Immunology

CASE
97

CASE 98

The patient with recurrent infection

A simulated patient with a history of recurrent infection is sometimes used to test the student's ability to discriminate between the various forms of immunodeficiency and their underlying causes.

? Causes

Primary immunodeficiency states are rare, but secondary immunodeficiency states are much more common.

Clinical features

The pattern, site and course of the infections that occur in an individual patient often give important clues to the most likely underlying cause or type of immunodeficiency state:

1 **Recurrent abscesses.** This suggests a defect in the non-specific phagocytic defence system, especially the neutrophils. A defect in neutrophil number, movement (chemotaxis), or ability to ingest (phagocytosis) or kill bacteria will lead to recurrent abscess formation. The latter may also occur as a result of chronic exposure to a pathogenic staphylococcal organism.

2 **Recurrent sinus and chest infection.** This suggests a defect in either antibody production (eg hypogammaglobulinaemia) or cilial movement (eg Kartagener's syndrome).

3 **Recurrent viral or fungal infection.** These infections occur in patients with a defect in the cell-mediated immune system.

4 **Bacterial, viral and fungal infections.** These infections occurring in an infant, together with a history of failure to thrive, suggest either severe combined immunodeficiency disease (SCID) or congenital human immunodeficiency virus (HIV) infection. In adults, acquired immunodeficiency syndrome (AIDS) would be the most likely cause (see Case 99).

5 **Same-site infection.** This should raise suspicion of some structural or functional abnormality which is predisposing to infection (eg a bronchogenic

CASE 98

neoplasm of the right middle lobe bronchus will result in recurrent right middle lobe infections; left vesico-ureteric reflux predisposes to recurrent left-sided pyelonephritis).

6 **Same-organism infection.** Repeated infections occurring over a period of months or years, but with an identical organism each time, would suggest that either the patient or a close contact is a chronic carrier of that organism (eg culture of swabs taken from bacterial carriage sites – nose, throat, axillae and groin – of a patient with recurrent skin abscesses or their spouse/partner often reveals a pathogenic staphylococcal organism identical to those isolated from the abscesses).

Primary immunodeficiency disorders

Because the immune system is essential for survival, it has evolved a variety of mechanisms to ensure that defects rarely occur. Serious primary immunodeficiency disorders result in death at an early age. Most of these disorders are inherited (mainly X-linked), and their prevalence in the population is extremely low – due to the fact that without treatment patients either die before reaching reproductive age or are infertile.

However, the student should have a knowledge of the major primary immuno-deficiency disorders. These can be summarised as follows:

1 Barriers – abnormal cilial function (eg Kartagener's syndrome).

2 Phagocytes:
- neutropenia
- Impaired motility
- impaired phagocytosis
- impaired bacterial killing (eg chronic granulomatous disease)
- Wiskott-Aldrich syndrome.

3 Complement system:
- selective deficiency states.

4 Antibody-mediated:
- selective IgA deficiency
- X-linked hypogammaglobulinaemia
- common variable immunodeficiency.

5 Cell-mediated:
- DiGeorge's syndrome

Immunology

CASE
98

- ataxia telangiectasia.

6. Both antibody- and cell-mediated:

- severe combined immunodeficiency disease (SCID).

Secondary immunodeficiency disorders

These are much more common causes of severe or recurrent infection. By far the commonest cause worldwide is HIV infection. This RNA retrovirus infects and destroys helper T lymphocytes which are necessary for controlling both cell-mediated and antibody-mediated immune responses (see Case 99).

The main causes of secondary immunodeficiency disorders or recurrent infections are as follows:

1 HIV infection

2 Drugs:

- cytotoxic drugs

- corticosteroids

- drugs which can cause bone marrow suppression as a side effect.

3 Underlying malignancy

4 Malnutrition

5 Major organ failure (eg renal or hepatic failure)

6 Ionising radiation.

In general, however, anything that causes defective functioning of the non-specific defence mechanisms (eg physical and chemical barriers, non-specific phagocytic cells and the complement components) or any disease process, drug or toxin which affects antibody production or lymphocyte number or function will predispose to bacterial or viral and fungal infection.

CASE
98

Immunology

CASE 99

Human immunodeficiency virus infection and AIDS

This major threat to human health is causing a global pandemic. All medical students and young doctors would be expected to have a good working knowledge of the condition. It could be encountered at a history-taking or data interpretation station where antibody levels and T lymphocyte subset results are available.

Definition

Acquired immunodeficiency syndrome (AIDS) is a secondary immunodeficiency disorder in which helper T lymphocyte depletion occurs as a result of infection with the RNA human immunodeficiency virus (HIV).

Clinical features

This condition mainly affects young adults and children born to mothers who are infected with HIV. The virus is present within lymphocytes, which are present in all bodily fluids, and infection is spread by sexual contact, blood or blood products, and can occur during childbirth or breastfeeding.

Because the current pandemic appears to have started in the male homosexual population, this group remains a major at-risk population. However, heterosexual and perinatal transmission is causing a major healthcare problem.

Seroconversion illness

After significant exposure to HIV, 50–80% of patients develop a glandular fever-like illness with sore throat, fever, cervical lymphadenopathy, malaise and muscle aches. This usually resolves within 2–3 weeks, but by this time most patients will have seroconverted (ie developed anti-HIV antibodies in their serum).

Asymptomatic phase

Following seroconversion the virus resides within a variety of cells, slowly replicating, eventually destroying the cell and infecting other cells which express the CD4+ cell-surface receptor (mainly found on helper T lymphocytes). At this time the patient is asymptomatic and clinical examination is normal. The only indication of infection is the presence of anti-HIV antibody.

Immunology

CASE
99

Persistent generalised lymphadenopathy

After a period of time (usually less than two years after HIV infection), the patient develops enlargement of lymph nodes which persists for more than three months and for which no other underlying cause can be found. Node enlargement is often symmetrical, and although it can occur at any lymph-node region, it most often affects the cervical, submandibular and axillary regions. In 25% of cases, splenomegaly can be detected on examination of the abdomen.

AIDS-related complex (ARC)

After some time, and with the partial immune deficiency that occurs when helper T lymphocyte depletion develops, the patient begins to develop constitutional symptoms. These include the following:

- intermittent or continuous fever
- weight loss
- night sweats
- diarrhoea
- lymphadenopathy.

At this stage the patient may have symptoms and signs of oral *Candida* infection. Investigations show a low CD4+ (helper T cell) count in the peripheral blood.

Acquired immunodeficiency syndrome (AIDS)

This is the final stage of HIV infection, when both the antibody- and cell-mediated immune systems fail to protect the individual. When the number of helper T cells falls below a critical level, the functioning of both types of specific immune response fails, resulting in the following conditions:

1 **Opportunistic infection.** Organisms that are normally non-pathogenic start to cause disease. Especially common are chest infections caused by *Pneumocystis carinii* (a protozoal organism), fungal infections (eg *Cryptococcus*) or atypical mycobacterial organisms (eg *Mycobacterium avium intracellulare*). Protozoal infection of the gastrointestinal tract, especially *Cryptosporidium* infection, causes episodes of profuse watery diarrhoea which can lead to severe dehydration and electrolyte abnormalities.

2 **Tumour development.** Cell-mediated immunity is important in anti-tumour surveillance. Patients with AIDS are especially susceptible to the development of Kaposi's sarcoma, non-Hodgkin's lymphoma and squamous-cell carcinomas.

CASE
99

3 **Central nervous system disorders.** Opportunistic infection of the central
nervous system is a common manifestation, especially with toxoplasmosis.
The human immunodeficiency virus also directly infects glial cells, and this
can cause a form of encephalopathy or progressive multifocal
leukoencephalopathy. The end stage of either is progressive cerebral atrophy
with features of a rapidly progressive presenile dementia.

Virtually any organism can cause infection. The major infective and other
manifestations are listed in Table 16.

Table 16 Common features of AIDS

Chest infection	*Pneumocystis carinii*
	Mycobacterium avium intracellulare
Gastrointestinal features	Oral and oesophageal candidiasis
	Hairy leukoplakia
	Cytomegalovirus oesophageal ulcers
	Cryptosporidiosis
	Cytomegalovirus hepatitis
Skin disorders	Kaposi's sarcoma
	Herpes zoster
	Squamous-cell carcinoma
Neurological features	Brain toxoplasmosis
	Herpes simplex encephalopathy
	Primary lymphoma of central nervous system
	Multifocal leukoencephalopathy
	Cerebral atrophy
Haemotological features	Leucopenia
	Non-Hodgkin's lymphoma
	Persistent lymphadenopathy
	Thrombocytopenia

Immunology

CASE
99

Investigations

A full blood picture usually shows a reduction in the total white cell count, mainly due to a decrease in the number of lymphocytes. T-lymphocyte subset analysis reveals a reduction in the number of helper T cells (CD4+ cells), with an inversion of the ratio of helper cells to suppressor cells (CD8+ cells). Normally the CD4+:CD8+ ratio is 2:1, whereas in patients with AIDS it is 1:2.

Immunoglobulins

Although patients with AIDS show impairment of specific antibody production, they usually have raised levels of IgG. This is due to the fact that before the immunodeficiency state develops they have had recurrent infections which stimulated antibody production. Only in the late stages of AIDS is the IgG level low.

HIV antibody and antigen tests

Within 2–3 weeks of HIV infection, serum antibodies can be detected in the patient, and these remain positive until late in the disease process. Viral antigen, especially the viral core antigen P24, can be detected by polymerase chain reaction (PCR) assays from an early stage of the disease. Before testing for HIV, it is important to make sure that the patient is fully informed of the implications of finding a positive result, and their full informed consent must be obtained before testing is carried out. Also, all blood samples, body fluids and biopsy material from patients with suspected HIV infection must be handled with great caution. Healthcare and laboratory staff must adhere to strict guidelines to prevent needlestick injury or exposure to potentially infectious material.

Treatment and management

Psychological and emotional support is extremely important, both at the time of diagnosis and at all stages of treatment. Patients and their close contacts will require counselling about prevention of spread of the disease.

Specific treatment is aimed at the clinical manifestations which the patient may show at the time of presentation, followed by the use of drugs which interfere with the replicative cycle of HIV (reverse transcriptase inhibitors) or the molecular biological steps needed for virus proliferation. Using combinations of these various drugs, virus replication can be inhibited and the disease process slowed down or brought to a halt. Much effort is being devoted to the development of an effective vaccine for this condition. To date, public health measures (health education) have been effective in altering behaviour (eg use of condoms, promotion of 'safe sex' measures, advice to drug addicts about the risks of sharing needles or syringes, etc).

**CASE
99**

CASE 100
Giant-cell arteritis and polymyalgia rheumatica

These conditions must be considered in any patient with a history of headache, as they commonly cause inflammation of the temporal arteries or muscle stiffness.

Giant-cell arteritis

 ### Definition

This is a form of vasculitis that affects medium-sized and large arteries and which most commonly affects the temporal arteries of the scalp. On histological examination, mononuclear inflammatory infiltration of the arterial wall and giant cell formation are seen.

Clinical features

Patients (usually over the age of 60 years) may have non-specific features of malaise and low-grade fever. If the temporal arteries are involved, the patient develops a unilateral or bilateral throbbing headache over the affected area of the scalp. On examination the arteries are thickened and tender. Involvement of arteries to the muscles of mastication can result in jaw claudication when the patient chews. Involvement of branches of the ophthalmic artery can result in ischaemic optic neuritis, which causes pain in the eye together with blurring of vision. A more serious complication is sudden blindness due to necrotising arteritis.

The condition often occurs in association with polymyalgia rheumatica (see below).

Investigations

The erythrocyte sedimentation rate (ESR) is usually > 100 mm/hour. Temporal artery biopsy shows characteristic mononuclear inflammation with giant cells.

Treatment

Patients respond to steroid therapy, and treatment should be started as soon as possible to reduce the risk of blindness. Initially the patient should be given prednisolone 60 mg daily, gradually decreasing over a period of weeks to a

Immunology

CASE
100

maintenance dose, which relieves the symptoms and results in a reduction in the ESR to within the normal range. Treatment should be continued for two years, after which 50% of patients will be cured and require no further therapy. However, 50% will develop a recurrence of their symptoms, often preceded by a rise in the ESR, and if this occurs corticosteroid therapy should be reintroduced.

Polymyalgia rheumatica

Definition

This condition is often associated with giant-cell arteritis, but can occur alone. It causes muscle stiffness of the shoulder girdle muscles. It may be used in a history-taking station for physical examination of a real or simulated patient.

Clinical features

Polymyalgia rheumatica is more common in women than in men, and rarely occurs in patients under the age of 55 years. The patient develops muscle stiffness and discomfort in the region of their shoulders, upper arms and neck. They have difficulty in raising their arms above their head, and start to experience difficulty dressing themselves or combing their hair.

On examination, the muscles are non-tender and muscle strength is normal, but the patient has stiffness on movement, with reduced ability to abduct the shoulder joint or raise their hands above the level of the shoulders. A history of headache and temporal artery tenderness may be present.

Investigations

The ESR is usually elevated (in the region of 100 mm/hour or more in the first hour). Muscle enzymes (eg creatine kinase) are normal.

Treatment

There is a dramatic and rapid improvement with corticosteroid therapy. Prednisolone 40 mg daily should be given for 2–4 weeks, and thereafter a gradual reduction to a maintenance dose of less than 15 mg daily is usually possible. The maintenance dose is determined by the patient's symptoms and the ESR. The aim of therapy is to keep the patient symptom-free and the ESR within the normal range (ie < 25 mm/hour).

Treatment is usually required for at least two years, after which it can be discontinued in 50% of patients. In patients who have a relapse of symptoms, long-term maintenance therapy is necessary.

Cardiovascular disorders

CASE 100

Index

Locators are by case number

PASTEST –
DEDICATED TO YOUR SUCCESS

PasTest has been publishing books for medical students and doctors for over 30 years. Our extensive experience means that we are always one step ahead when it comes to knowledge of current trends in undergraduate exams.

We use only the best authors, which enables us to tailor our books to meet your revision needs. We incorporate feedback from candidates to ensure that our books are continually improved.

This commitment to quality ensures that students who buy PasTest books achieve successful exam results.

Delivery to your door

With a busy lifestyle, nobody enjoys walking to the shops for something that may or may not be in stock. Let us take the hassle and deliver direct to your door. We will dispatch your book within 24 hours of receiving your order.

How to Order:

www.pastest.co.uk

To order books safely and securely online, shop at our website.

Telephone: +44 (0)1565 752000 Fax: +44 (0)1565 650264

For priority mail order and have your credit card to hand when you call.

Write to us at:

PasTest Ltd
FREEPOST
Haig Road
Parkgate Industrial Estate
Knutsford
WA16 7BR

PASTEST BOOKS FOR MEDICAL STUDENTS

PasTest are the specialists in study guides and revision courses for medical qualifications. For over 30 years we have been helping doctors to achieve their potential. The PasTest range of books for medical students includes:

Essential Skills Practice for OSCEs in Medicine   1 904627 38 2
David McCluskey

100 Clinical Cases and OSCEs in Surgery   1 904627 00 5
Noel Aherne, Enda McDermott, Arnold D K Hill

OSCEs for Medical Students, 2nd edition, Volume 1   1 901198 04 9
Adam Feather, Ramanathan Visvanathan, John SP Lumley

OSCEs for Medical Students, 2nd edition, Volume 2   1 901198 05 7
Adam Feather, Ramanathan Visvanathan, John SP Lumley

OSCEs for Medical Students, 2nd edition, Volume 3   1 904627 11 0
Adam Feather, Ramanathan Visvanathan, John SP Lumley,
Jonathan Round

EMQs for Medical Students Volume 1   1 901198 65 0
Adam Feather et al

EMQs for Medical Students Volume 2   1 901198 69 3
Adam Feather et al

EMQs for Medical Students: Practice Papers, Volume 3   1 904627 07 2
Adam Feather et al

Essential MCQs for Medical Finals, Second edition   1 901198 20 0
Rema Wasan, Delilah Hassanally, Balvinder Wasan

Essential MCQs for Surgical Finals, Second edition   1 901198 15 4
Delilah Hassanally, Rema Singh

Essential MCQs in Clinical Pharmacology   1 901198 32 4
Delilah Hassanally, Rema Singh